The Invinsible Observer

by Roosevelt Bwalya Kasonso

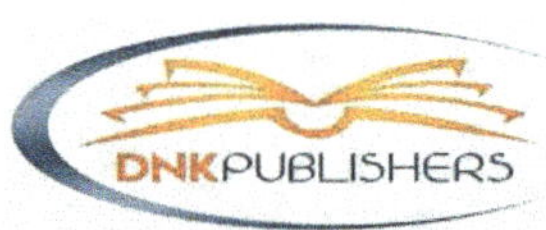

First Published 2022 by

DNK Brand and Publishers

24 Chimanga Road, Lusaka, Zambia

dnkpublishers@gmail.com

Contact: +260 979 961 647

©Roosevelt Bwalya Kasonso

Mobile: +260 97 3452433

E-mail: rooseveltkas@gmail.com

Table of contents

Introduction

I was inspired to write this book by the journey I have travelled through life, facing different challenges and experiences, some of them positive, others negative which have shaped who I am today. My past does not describe who I am, but without all the failures, disappointments and addictions, I wouldn't be better than I was yesterday. So I believe the process of being shaped in life through experiences both negative and positive is very necessary, and from the many people, I am one person who has seriously benefited from learning from my mistakes. I have grown wiser and through the troublesome moments, I have been made stronger and even through my lowest moments in life, I have gained clarity and an understanding that we have purpose and there is a meaning to our existence. My journey through life has been dramatic from struggling with addictions, some wild experiences, encounters with the law and some life threatening events. I am glad to say I don't regret any part of it because there was a purpose for me to have gone through whatever I went through, and I believe every part of the journey is a necessary experience. I am also glad to be a life guide who people can run to for advice on various life challenges. I am now content with the man I am and I believe everything in life happens at God's time because it's all part of God's plan. As humans, we are all unique in our individual ways and at some point, we might have all struggled with something in life. It might not only be an addiction but after getting out of the depths of hell, I would like to provide a light for someone in the dark, I would like to give some hope to someone who is lost and show them we do recover no matter how far you might go in the wrong direction, you can always turn back. I have personally struggled with multiple addictions in life and I have put up this book as a guide to anyone who might want to get out of a similar situation or help someone who is struggling with something. I firstly want to thank

Mum who has been an inspiration and gave me a green light to go out become the author of my destiny, I want to thank you for always being an anchoring pillar in my life and always believing that I had whatever it takes to make it in life and for everyone who encouraged me to turn my writing into a reality. This includes my brothers, Kayamba, Muntala, Mulusa and my sister Mollisa. Without forgetting my late aunty, Judy. May her soul rest in eternal peace. I am grateful for her encouragement and I also want to dedicate this book to everyone fighting a silent battle with hope of improving their livelihood.

My brothers and sisters in recovery, and my colleagues, Madam Indra, Madam Yuma, Madam Alice, Madam Alpha, Mr Lubanda, Mr Mwelwa, Mr Kalaluka, you always have a special place in my heart. I also want to thank the director of the Great North Road Group of Companies Doctor Rozious Siatwambo for being a great mentor who has always echoed the words that you cannot work under a great man and still remain the same and always encouraged everyone to grow in their individual capacity. I want to also thank Mr. Daniel Kabani for being part of my journey as an inspirational guide, Madam Precious, Madam Eunice, my lecturer Madam Malipa and many more I have not mentioned.

The title of this book, *The Invisible Observer,* is taken from the three dimensions which I have used in my approach to addiction recovery. One is from the addicts point of view, I talk about my experiences in various addictions as an abuser from my initial use of marijuana, heroin, diazepam, alcohol and codeine to the point where I had finally hit rock bottom and I was left with no choice because it was now a matter of life and death, and the only way out was to go clean. I also approach recovery addiction from the therapeutic point of view as a counselor or a sponsor and how I have been a light to someone in the dark, a friend, a colleague and an ear to anyone who is willing to talk, and above all, I am glad to be a shoulder to lean on for anyone who has fallen and struggling to pick himself up. I also take a look at addiction recovery from a family member's point of view who has seen a brother, a child, an uncle, a nephew, a niece, a friend, a neighbor, a parent or any loved one struggling with this disease of addiction. I have come to understand that there is always hope to recover from any addiction as long as one recognizes it in time and accepts.

The first part of this book talks about my personal struggles and how I started out with the smoking and the progression of addiction through the different phases of life and circumstances others of which might have made the situation worse. The first part also highlights how I initially tried out substances and the transition of addiction from my early teenage years to also switching addictions and the circumstances that made this addiction grow, not forgetting the environmental factors which help reinforce some of these compulsions. Later in the chapters, I have touched on why addiction is not because of poor choices and lack of will power but as one digs deeper into the later chapters, you will clearly understand how the brain gets compromised with the body at large becoming automatically wired and making it hard for one to break out of addiction even when willing. I have also shared my life experiences of friends and family members who struggled with depression and addiction, others, are gone and may their souls rest in peace while others are still struggling in the hope of one day breaking free from the different stressors that come with society on a daily basis. I would also like to mention that issues of mental health need to be given serious attention by all the stakeholders.This includes society and the people in authority. Every individual is vulnerable to becoming depressed if they don't take good care of their mental health, while others already have underlying health conditions or chronic disease which society has stigmatized. I would also like to note that no one is immune to the daily stressors, frustrations, failures and disappointments that come with life and so there comes the need for society to make our environment as friendly as possible by educating everyone on how they can handle different pressures that come with life.

1

How It Started

I got exposed to smoking marijuana when I was 16 years of age. I was in grade 10 at Chililabombwe Secondary School. I used to hang around with people who were much way older than me. I wanted to fit in with this group of friends and just being young around that age, I was very prone to peer pressure and as a teenager, there is always an urge to try out different experiences as one is trying to find their true identity. So I was trying out different lifestyles. I tried marijuana for the first time out of curiosity because the guys I used to hang around with where regular users and I sometimes imagined how it would feel like to be jade as they used call the marijuana high. Though the initial experience was not so positive, I kept on using so as not to be looked upon as a coward or a kembo in the group as they say on the street. Around that time, I had a childhood passion for music to become a rap star like the American musicians we used watch on the then popular music channel called channel O. We would smoke and go to our makeshift bedroom studio where we would spend the whole day playing back radio cassettes tapes to write down lyrics and mime to the songs.

I was a fan and follower of the wrong model type the then gangsters the 2 pac shakur's, snoop dogg, Eminem and many more old school rappers. At that age, being a gangster was the thing and using drugs was cool like the models we looked up to. Little did I know that the lifestyle was slowly throwing me into problems. I continued with the regular smoking and bad company and as the years went by, I became hooked on the marijuana and become fully dependent on the substance to an extent where I would experience all kinds of withdraws in forms of physical and emotional discomfort. This was about the time Dad passed away and we had to relocate from a *Mayadi* or residential household arrangement to a *komboni* or ghetto arrangement. We shifted to a compound where the care takers of the house we were renting from were drug pushers. Due to availability of substances, the drug use increased. This became my new normal due to easy access. As time went by, I spent my teenage years living this rebellious lifestyle characterized by drug and alcohol abuse. My academic performance declined as I lost focus on school and was usually associated with the worst behaved kids at school, notoriously known as the dagga smokers and bad company. I often had problems with the school authorities and on several occasions would be caught smoking marijuana on the school premises or stealing books from the storeroom to sell to other pupils. We also had a routine of going out of bounds by jumping the school wall fence only to waste those school days smoking marijuana and drinking buckets of chibuku in the nearby community tarvens.

These untimely escapades continued into the exam year which really drove me of course, and this played a big role in getting poor grades during my grade 12 secondary school results. I later switched my addictions and got into alcohol which also took another drain on my life, I started drinking as a social drinker and as the drinking become more regular, I became dependent on alcohol and eventually became alcoholic. My alcoholic journey was characterized by a negative lifestyle, disappointments, unprogressive behaviors, crime and self-sabotaging behaviors. I kept on with the drinking and thugging lifestyle which on several occasions got me on the wrong side of the law for cases like criminal trespassing, loitering at awkward hours, stock theft, obtaining money by false pretense and being found in position of stolen property. I got used to being locked up in jail and became an expert in conning my way out of the prison cells. As I continued on this destructive path, I entertained a wrong company of friends, among them were drug dealers, criminals, thieves and junkies of whom most had lost direction and had no plans for the future and for most of them going to prison was an achievement which was deserving of praise.

It is a very common lifestyle for the majority of the youth who wake up every morning with no hope for the future, the only goal is to meet up in bars every morning and drinking and blaming the government for their laziness to break out of their comfort zone ane embark on a job search. As I continued on this destructive path, I created a prison within my mind which continued landing me in the same circle and eventually led me into depression. As this lifestyle continued, I reached a stage where I started drinking my life away and thinking it was worthless to be alive.

Rejection, Failure and Depression

There are a lot of people out there who have become frustrated with life and contemplate suicide because they keep on being disappointed and society has also demonized them for being failures. Eventually, they sink into feelings of rejections. A few months earlier, I had lost my cousin back home in the village after he went through a depressive period. He was sponsored to do an electrical and electronics engineering program in Malaysia for 3 years after which he come back without any qualification but just an accent. The some Asian countries a student's visa only allows one to strictly do school work and no part time jobs as opposed to the Western world where one can also do side jobs to supplement their finances. This meant that survival was entirely dependent on handouts from the family who at that time had the financial muscle. However, nomatter how financially affluent one might be, there is always a strain on the sources of money especially when one is solely dependent on business, the whole cost comes to making sacrifices at the expense of growing your business. So when my cousin came back home after 3 years abroad, there was that excitement upon arrival, like it was the return of the prodigal son though the appearance, the accent, the slang, the fluency, the dress code could all be depicted from afar that this lad had crossed the oceans as I have learned in a recent times that most people who have had a chance to live overseas come with some sort of attitude with Western influenced cultural values.

Well, as the honeymoon period winged off, the true reality of the situation kicked in, my cousins school was a total failure as there was no certification, diploma or degree whatsoever to show for the past three years in the diaspora. This was received with frustration especially from his father, the financier. Coming to terms with the reality of the situation was no easy thing. There was an element of rejection from the entire family as he was now considered a failed project and a loss of money invested but as this continued, he resorted to excessive drinking to dispel the dissonance he was experiencing as he also failed to come to terms with reality. He unnoticeably went into depression and every time he was reminded of school affair, his depression got worse.

The condition got him to a point of contemplating suicide and on this fateful day, they had an argument with his father and little did anyone know that he had already bought a bottle of doom, a pesticide, and this time around he never hesitated to take a sip. I woke up the following day with one thing pressing on my mind. I hadn't been in contact with my cousin, so I reached out to give him a shout but hIs phone went unanswered. Rejection is an inevitable part of life. But it can still be hurtful, even when you're in a great headspace. If you experience rejection while dealing with depression, it can be even harder to navigate. People with depression often feel hopeless and worthless, and being rejected can echo those emotions. Rejection is associated with increased substance abuse and risk of suicide, in particular, social isolation and family discord are directly linked to elevated risks of suicide.

Addiction

Addiction is a disease involving continued use of a substance despite serious substance-related problems such as loss of control over use, health problems or negative social consequences.

Addiction is when your body gets used to doing something so well that it surpasses your mind. Addiction is simply a compulsion to engage in any activity resulting in dependency. This happens when the body becomes good at doing something more than the mind, even amongst adverse effects one still clings to the activity when it is clearly evident that this activity is harmful or is negatively impacting one's life but they do it anyway.

I had kept on using marijuana and alcohol despite its negative impact it had on my life, there were several occasions when things would become so bad like at one time a police officer visited our house to carry out an inspection after our neighbour's house had been broken into and a disco music system was stolen. I usually had the habit of dropping seeds of marijuana in a flower pot whenever making a joint.

The flower pots were always watered so at some point, the seeds took root and a plant of cannabis started growing. I noticed it at some point but I entertained the idea and convincing myself that it would grow into a high quality weed. However, on this fateful day, the man in uniform noticed a rare type of flower which had grown and he easily identified it as cannabis.

Outside the house was my younger brother, so the uniformed police officer asked if there was any older male child and my brother immediately come to call me from my room where I was listening to some reggae music by Bob Marley. I was also surprised to hear that a police officer was asking for me, so I went outside to meet him and he pointed at the cannabis plant and asked if I had any idea what it was, as I nodded my head in agreement that I knew the plant, he immediately got a pair of handcuffs and suggested I accompany him to the police station and give statement to the drug enforcement officers about being found with a banned psychotropic substance. Little was I aware that letting such a substance grow in a domestic environment was a breach of the law, and if it wasn't for my uncle's immediate intervention who offered the police officer some money to just get rid of the evidence and forget that the incident ever happened, with an assurance that I would never be careless with such incriminating substances in the future again, I would have been taken away. It is also a characteristic of addiction for one to become careless and leave substances lying around where they can easily be discovered as they progress into risky use.

Functional Addicts

A functioning addict is a person who is struggling with substance abuse but can outwardly project normalcy. Functional addicts take great care to avoid looking like people who have lost control of their lives. They are good at hiding their problems. They are fearful that if found out, their reputation and career will suffer. Functional addicts continue to hold down a job. Many enjoy great professional success. Also functioning addicts usually maintain active social lives. They can successfully hide their addictions from even closest friends and family members.

However, because functioning addicts appear normal to their friends, family, and colleagues, they are at a great risk from the dangers of drug and alcohol abuse. Often times, the addiction is discovered too late, and a functioning addict becomes the victim of an overdose. Many functional addicts can sustain a relationship for an extended period, causing significant damage to their health, relationships, and financial status.

There are many functional addicts in society ranging from doctors, nurses, lawyers, police officers, teachers, lecturers, politicians, enterprenuers and engineers only to mention a few. At some point in our journey through life, we have all been groomed or attended to by a functional addict and they are usually experts in what they do.

Back in the day when I was at Copperstone University persuing my diploma in Electrical and electronics engineering, I had a lecturer by the name of Mr. Limbubu who used to tutor me in engineering drawing and drinking tujilijili course. He had studied in Russia and I understand the weather allows people to drink whiskey for breakfast or maybe people who have had an opportunity to study in Russia just love to justify their drinking habits. It was the norm for my lecturer every morning before class to first drink about 500 ml of whiskey in order for him to be his normal self and able to lecture. His class was always packed and interesting, at one point it become a routine for him to call for me first thing in the morning and send me to buy 6 satchets of Tujilijili of which he would share two with me before he would take our class into a lecture. He knew his job very well as every time he taught us, he would say he was not preparing us for the exams but was preparing us to go and do the actual work in the industry, sad to say he developed liver problems and other health complications as a result of excessive alcohol consumption which led to his death, may his soul rest in eternal peace.

It is a fact that people with addiction problems know they have to stay employed to pay for their substance abuse. The signs of addiction may be visible in the work place, but colleagues and supervisors tend to look the other way as long as the person is fulfilling their work responsibilities. Addiction affects many aspects of a person's life, including health, social life and finances. It takes a terrible toll on families. But family members accommodate a person's addiction for years, allowing them to continue as a functioning addict until they eventually get fed up.

Addiction doesn't discriminate. It can affect the young and old, the rich and poor, the educated and uneducated. But the key characteristic of a functioning addict is the ability to maintain stable and successful careers.

High Stress Occupations That Are At Risk Of Functional Addiction:

Law enforcement officers: The daily stresses of the job and various threatening and disturbing events can push law enforcement officers towards using illicit substances as a coping mechanism. Drug and alcohol addiction in law enforcement officers is very high. A lot of alcohol and drug abuse is very common both in the police and military service personnel which in most cases is masked under their uniforms. It is easy to notice though, but just getting our men in service to introspect themselves is very hard unless usually when their jobs are threatened. The problem also comes in because even the work environment becomes an enabling factor where they are in constant confrontations with criminals.

Lawyers: More than 20 percent of lawyers or attorneys report harmful and potentially addictive drinking patterns. Depression, anxiety and stress are also common among lawyers, conditions that often concur with substance abuse.

Healthcare personnel: Doctors and nurses work in high stress environments. Also, health personnel have easy access to powerful prescription drugs.

Business executives: Intense, high-pressure work environments and long hours can drive business executives towards drugs and alcohol. In particular, these tend to use smart drugs to enhance their concentration and enhance creativity.

Bus drivers and Public Transport Officers: Because of the stress that comes with working long hours and the environmental factors in the stations where one is required to be aggressive in winning customers, most drivers and conductors or public transport officers usually actively resort to alcohol or other drugs to boost their confidence levels to deal with the pressure that comes with their work.

Identifying A Functional Addict

High functioning addicts can show up for work every day whilst struggling with substance abuse. And if addiction treatment and drug or alcohol rehab are not begun early enough, they are at a high risk of physical and psychological harm. That is why it is important to know the signs of a functional addiction. Here are the signs to look out for:

Denial: Many functional addicts are not convinced they have a problem. *"I work so hard, I deserve to have fun." "I drink to unwind after a day's hard work."* The denials can sound quite reasonable, but in truth, no job, however stressful, should require habitual drug or alcohol use.

I remember a time back when I was in Solwezi, I was working at Kasanshi Copper and Gold mines as a security guard under Group 4 Security company where this time I was fired from work for drinking on duty, I had developed a habit of smuggling alcohol and drugs to work especially when doing night shifts. It is a trend for most security guards who work in the night to either report for work drunk or carry alcohol to work which is used as a cusion against the cold or some form of courage used to brave through the night while everyone else is sleeping. We used to guard in the most dangerous beats on the mines which were targets for thieves who were interested in the solar panels and heavy duty batteries. So alcohol and drugs was a friend that would walk you through the night.

However, the habit become normalized as at times we would link up with other guards from different sites to share the alcohol, marijuana and cigarates. On this fateful morning as I was knocking off, I was summoned to the commander's officer to collect my bus pass, as I entered the office which was full of other high ranking officers, they smelled the strong whiskey as I passed and immediately subjected me to a breatharizer which detected the alcohol. I was instantly put on forced leave and eventually relieved of my duties as a security officer. The days that followed got me into feeling frustrated, disappointed and full of shame and guilt which led me into abusing more alcohol. It was at this point that my neighbor, a lady who worked as a cleaner at Solwezi General Hospital asked if I would be interested in a job at the hospital. She informed me of an internal memo in which they required a mortuary attendant with no work experience. She also mentioned that most mortuary attendants were allowed to drink on duty and there were also extra allowances with every corpse that required a post mortem. I plainly rejected this offer as my worry was my mental and psychological health after I would have left that job.

Excuses: Functional addicts often make excuses and chalk up their drug or alcohol use as standard behavior in their profession. They use their professional success to justify illicit substance use.

Isolation: Functional addicts become more and more consumed by their addiction as time goes on. They put relationships, work, family, and community on the back burner. As the addiction progresses, addicts are only interested in one thing – getting their next hit.

Enabling relationships: People who are functional addicts often seek validation from others like themselves. It's not uncommon for certain professions to have enabling environments where people encourage each other to indulge in bad behavior.

Unexplained financial losses: Addictive substances do not come cheap. Even though functional addicts may maintain a façade of normalcy, they may be unable to hide large sums of missing money from family members. Substance use disorders can quickly escalate and make finances unmanageable. This should be a red flag to loved ones that something is going on behind the scenes.

Help For a Functional Addict

Alcohol and drug abuse impact a person's judgment and alertness at work, their relationships at home, their health, and their finances. Yet people with substance use disorders become preoccupied with obtaining and using illicit drugs. Many addicts undertake illegal activities such as selling drugs to other people, to fund their drug habit. Functional addicts are very good at covering their tracks and hiding their struggles with alcohol or drugs. Functional addicts are especially at risk from the dangers of substance abuse because their addiction can go unnoticed for a very long time. That is why it is important to be vigilant for drug abuse and alcoholism in colleagues, friends and family members. A proactive approach to drug and alcohol addiction treatment can help functional addicts the help they need before it is too late.

Why People Get Addicted

Addiction causes changes in the brain's structure and functioning. It is not caused by poor will power or character flaws. Addiction can grow slowly and isn't always easy to see, many people with addiction continue to function in some parts of their life but have problems in other areas.

Just as the transition into addiction is gradual, the signs also begin gradually like first losing control over substance use which may be a drug of one's choice or alcohol. This can start by one using more of the substance than intended, to having difficulties in reducing substance use and it also goes from one spending significant time planning on how to obtain substances to having strong desire and craving to use. There are many problems that come with addiction, but despite the worst life threatening one's, the user is always blinded to how it negatively it affects him.

There is a wide variety of addictions ranging from substances like coffee, coca-cola, alcohol, drugs like heroin, marijuana, cocaine, codeine, methamphetamine, valium, shisha, cigarettes, insuko and prescription pills amongst the commonly abused. Other forms of addictions fall into pornography addiction, sex addiction, technology addiction like social media addiction and video games, eating disorders like food addiction, obsessive disorders like spiritual obsession, exercise obsession and work obsession and many more.

When any habit becomes an addiction, it is no longer a matter of choice or self-control but it has become a disease or an illness. So addiction is a progressive chronic illness whose reasons or conditions for use will differ from why they started in the first place. I started smoking marijuana when I was 16 years in my 10th grade. I used to hang around with friends who had already been exposed to drugs and they were comfortable with the habit. The more I was around this company of users, the more I started feeling the urge to try out and experiment and also to feel more part of the group. I one day asked the guys if I could take a pull from the blunt, at first I did not properly inhale the smoke but on the second pull, as the marijuana smoke passed out of my nostrils, I felt an elevated and distorted perception clouding my vision as I heard the sounds of nature becoming louder. I immediately convinced myself that this was an experience worth frequenting.

 I began to enjoy this activity and never wanted to miss any session. As I repeatedly indulged in the habit, I slowly built a tolerance were the quantity and frequency increased. In the shortest period of time I became friends with every reliable supplier of marijuana in my hood. Our trade ties became stronger as money was not the only currency since I would trade cloths, gadgets and at times steal relish for exchange with drugs. As I continued using these drugs, I could not function without the marijuana component. I had graduated into dependency, and it was also a way of coping from negative or elevated emotions. I also deceived myself believing it increased my creativity as an upcoming rap musician. The choice of role models in society has also a negative impact on the lifestyle of many youths as I looked up to the wrong role models in this world. I also won't run away from the fact that the presence of a male parent is key in a child's life as there was a void of not having a father figure to look up to, in the end falling prey to scavenging drug dealers.

Many people don't understand why or how people become addicted to drugs or alcohol. They may mistakenly think that those who use drugs lack moral principles or willpower and they could stop their drug use simply by choosing to. In reality, drug addiction is a complex disease, quitting usually takes more than good intentions or good will. Drugs can change the brain in ways that make quitting harder even for those who want to.

The initial decision to take drugs or alcohol is voluntary for most people, repeated substance use can lead to brain changes that challenge an addicted person's self-control and interfere with their ability to resist. These brain changes can be persistent which is why addiction is considered a relapsing disease. People in recovery are at increased risk of returning to active use even after years of not taking. This is because of the many stressors life presents and the ever existing triggers which differ from individual to individual.

Whenever a person does a new activity for the first time, a neural pathway is formed that links the new activity to the brain. The more one engages in this activity, the more it is reinforced and made stronger because the more these neurons will fire and wire together. So, even for any new habit, new neural connections are formed connecting to that new activity and the more it is done, the more it is reinforced such that even when one ceases to engage in this activity, the neural pathways still remain except they may not be as strong as one who is actively engaging. These neural pathways never disappear, so even for anyone who has struggled with any addiction, certain neural pathways connecting to these addictions were formed and never disappear nomatter how long they can stay away.

Whenever one experiences feelings of discomfort like anger, anxiety, boredom, fear, excitement and confusion, the body always wants an escape from these emotions, people will always resort to finding a way to cope with these emotions by either using substances like drugs or alcohol or any other activities to numb such feelings. When one uses this as a way to cope, they end up creating a prison in their mind that only acknowledges coping with substances as a path of least resistance to cope with stress, anxiety or any negative feeling. Whenever one is stressed, it is easy for their body to unconsciously push them to using substances because of the neural pathway that were created while engaging in these addictions. The body always chooses the path of least resistance to cope with stress, I remember I always opted to drinking alcohol or using drugs as a way of escaping any feeling of discomfort. This was my way of coping with stress, anger, anxiety, rejection even excitement and this is what has kept many people going in circles of addiction and even worse for others. It is the painful stomach crumbs, the junces, the anxiety and fear of withdraw that what keeps them locked in this mental prison of addiction.

Chemical Addiction

A Chemical addiction is a chronic, progressive and potentially fatal brain disease characterized by loss of control over use, denial and relapse. It is also characterized by continuous use of substance despite harmful and negative consequences.

Different chemicals affect different brains in different ways. Some people are attracted to substances from the first time they use them and find they need more. For other people, drugs or alcohol register negatively and they have no desire for more from the beginning.

A person's vulnerability to becoming addicted appears to depend on three factors.

1. Genetics – if an individual has relatives with a history of drugs or alcohol problems, it may indicate that they face a heightened risk of developing addictions themselves.
2. Environment – the circumstances within which a person grows up and lives their lives, including family, friends and peer pressure, stresses and inherent fears and insecurities can influence the risk of an individual misusing drugs or alcohol.
3. Age of first use – Science has found that the earlier a person starts to use alcohol or drugs, the greater the risk of developing an addiction.

- There are two components to chemical addictions, the brain and the chemicals. Once a chemical is introduced to the body and it makes its way to the brain, the interaction that occurs will determine the problems that may arise.

- Fundamentally, alcohol and drugs initially cause a reaction that the brain interprets positively. Most produce euphoria or a sense of relief from tension and stress.

- They can heighten a person's self-confidence, wellbeing and a person's feeling of being in control. They can also bring a welcome feeling of drowsiness and sleep.

- But alcohol and drugs, if misused, can also create a host of physical and emotional side effects that are detrimental, if not disastrous to the user.

- Past the obvious effects of misusing substances such as a person slurring their words and losing balance, addictive substances have emotional and intellectual consequences too.

- They can erode rational thinking to a point where behaviors that a person knows are dangerous such as driving a vehicle while drunk for example or becoming physically or verbally abusive to others seem to make sense.

- A brain under the influence of drugs or alcohol can be affected physically, emotionally, psychologically and spiritually by these substances.

- This is why it is often said that drugs and alcohol hijack the brain. The most commonly misused and abused substances are:

1. Alcohol – this drug is by far the most used and abused substance. It is legally purchased at the age of 21 and 18 in other places, it is heavily advertised and socially acceptable. It is also the number one gateway drug for the youth.

2. Opioids (heroin, morphine and codeine) – These drugs are available both legally and prescribed or illegal as street drugs. Morphine is the active component in heroin, also known on the street as volo or Tia white which is the cheapest and most addictive substance and can potentially get someone hooked even on being used for the first time. Its addictive quality is enhanced by adding dangerous chemicals like pesticides and battery acid to easily get someone addicted from their initial use.

3. Stimulants (cocaine, crack cocaine and amphetamines) – These stimulants create energy excitement and euphoria, and can also be highly addictive.

4. Depressants (prescribed sedatives, tranquilizers, benzodiazepines and valium) –These are accessed as prescribed medicines but excessive and long term use can lead to addiction. Sometimes misused in conjunction with other substances to enhance sensations of euphoria or relaxation.

5. Marijuana – this is a psychoactive drug from cannabis plant which has been used as a drug for recreational purposes and in various traditional medicines for centuries. Marijuana is dried leaves and flowers of the *cannabis sativa*. Many people try

out marijuana because of the main psychoactive ingredient, THC, which stimulates part of the brain that responds to pleasure, like food and sex. That unleashes a chemical called dopamine, which gives euphoria, a relaxed feeling. However, not everyone's experience with marijuana is pleasant, it can often leave one anxious, afraid, panicked or paranoid. Using marijuana may rise the chances for clinical depression or worsen the symptoms of any mental disorder one already has. When used in high doses, it makes one paranoid and lose touch with reality, making one hear and see things that are not there.

- As with other potentially addicting substances, the risk of dependency on marijuana appears to hinge on how the individual's brain interacts with the substance.

Signs And Symptoms Of Addiction

All addictions, whether to substances or to behaviors, involve physical or psychological processes. Each person's experience of addiction is slightly different, but there are generally some common symptoms to watch out for, including behavioral changes like lying, extreme changes in mood, and changing social groups, as well as physical symptoms like changes in weight, sleep and energy levels.

Common signs of addiction include:

- Changes in social groups, new and unusual friends, odd phone conversations.
- Financial problems
- Repeated unexplained outings, often with a sense of urgency
- Lying
- Secretiveness

- Stealing
- Stashes of drugs, often in small plastic, paper or foil packages
- Activities centering on the addiction in a way that negatively affects relationships, school and work
- A preoccupation with the addiction and spending a lot on time planning, engaging in, and recovering from the addictive behavior
- Changes in energy, such as being unexpectedly and extremely tired or energetic
- Difficulty cutting down or controlling the addictive behavior
- Extreme mood changes
- Physical changes including increased illness and changes in weight
- Sleeping a lot or less than usual, or at different times of the day or night
- Tolerance, which involves the need to engage in the addictive behavior more and more to get the desired effect
- Withdrawal, when the person does not take the substance or engage in the activity, and they experience unpleasant symptoms.

Symptoms of Specific Addictions

While there are signs and symptoms of a general nature, certain substances and behaviors can come with their own set of symptoms.

- Behaviors (gambling, exercise, sex, shopping): Behavioral addictions are characterized by compulsive behaviors that persist despite negative consequences.

- Depressants (alcohol, barbiturates, benzodiazepines):these medications slow the activity of central nervous system and slowed heartbeat and respiration, confusion, coma, and death.
- Opioids (pain killers, heroin, morphine): These substances decrease sensitivity to pain and produce strong cravings for opioids.
- Stimulants (caffeine, nicotine, amphetamines, methamphetamine, cocaine): These substances lead to high energy levels.

Complications & Comorbidities

Although drug use and addiction can happen at any time during a person's life, drug use typically starts in adolescence, a period when the first signs of mental illness commonly appear. During the transition to young adulthood (18 to 25 years), people with comorbid disorders need coordinated support to help them navigate potentially stessful changes in education, work and relationships.

The brain continues to develop through adolescence. Circuits that control executive functions such as decision making and impulse control are among the last to mature, which enhances vulnerability to drug use and the development of a substance use disorder, and it may be a risk factor for the later occurrence of other mental illnesses.

It is also true that having a mental disorder in childhood or adolescence can increase the risk of later drug use and the development of a substance use disorder. Some research has found that mental illness may precede a substance use disorder, suggesting that better diagnosis of youth mental illness may help reduce comorbidity. One study found that adolescent onset bipolar disorder confers a greater risk of subsequent substance use disorder compared to adult-onset bipolar disorder.

Three main-pathways can contribute to comorbidity between substance use disorders and mental illnesses.

1. Common risk factors can contribute to both mental illness and substance use and addiction.
2. Mental illness may contribute to substance use and addiction.
3. Substance use and addiction can contribute to the development of mental illness.

Both substance use disorders and other mental illnesses are caused by overlapping factors such as genetic and epigenetic vulnerabilities, issues with similar areas of the brain, and environmental influences such as early exposure to stress or trauma.

Certain mental disorders are established risk factors for developing a substance use disorder. It is commonly hypothesized that individuals with severe, mild, or even subclinical mental disorders may use drugs as a form of self-medication.

Behavioral Addictions

Most people understand addiction when it comes to a dependence on substances such as alcohol, nicotine, illicit drugs or even prescribed medications, but have a hard time with the concept of addictive behaviors.

Yet, it's possible to develop a behavioral addiction. In fact, people can get hooked on everything from gambling to sex to the internet.

Some activities are so normal, it is hard to believe people can become addicted to them. Yet the circle of addiction can still take over, making everyday life a struggle. People may seek out more and more opportunities to engage in the behavior. The desire to engage in the behavior becomes so strong that the individual continues to engage in the activity despite negative consequences.

In some cases, people can also experience withdrawal, including negative emotions and other symptoms, when they aren't able to engage in the activity.

Behavioral addictions have similar effects to substance addictions on relationships, which are often neglected in favor of the addictive behavior, undermining trust and putting pressure on partners and other family members to cover up and make up for difficulties arising from the addiction.

Signs that you have a Behavioral Addiction

Understanding the addictive process and the dangerous signs can help you tell the difference between addictive behavior, and normal behavior that's non-problematic.

Red flags include:

- Spending the majority of your time engaging in the behavior, thinking about or arranging to engage in the behavior, or recovering from the effects.
- Becoming dependent on the behavior as a way to cope with emotions and to feel normal.
- Continuing despite physical and/or mental harm.
- Having trouble cutting back despite wanting to stop
- Neglecting work, school, or family to engage in behavior more often.

- Experiencing symptoms of withdrawal (for example, depression or irritability) when trying to stop
- Minimizing or hiding the extent of the problem.

Some common behavioral addictions include:

- Exercise addiction
- Food addiction
- Gambling addiction
- Internet addiction
- Porn addiction
- Sex addiction
- Shopping addiction
- Tattoo addiction

Consequences of Addictions

Even when not specifically labelled as addictions, compulsive behaviors can lead to real problems in a person's life, functioning and relationships. These behaviors can create considerable distress and be difficult to change, even when the person wants to stop. These addictions usually result in losses that seem too great to bear, such as money problems or relationship problems. What had at one time seemed exciting and fulfilling becomes an embarrassing burden.

In truth, the consequences of drug addiction affect physical, mental, social and spiritual health often severely.

Physical Consequences

The physical consequences of addiction are perhaps the most obvious to the individual. Scrapes, bruises, track marks, lip burns, skin abscesses, disease (like HIV or Hepatitis C), increased tolerance, physical dependence and withdrawal symptoms are physical consequences of addiction.

Mental Consequences

Some of the mental consequences are depression, anxiety, mood swings and psychosis. While psychosis is usually a direct result of drug use, depression, anxiety and mood swings can be both a direct and indirect result and can persist after drug use has stopped. When a person suffers from addiction and also has a mental health disorder, whether it began before or after substance use, such a condition is called dual diagnosis. Dual diagnosis treatment is most effective in these cases.

Social Consequences

The social consequences of addiction are usually the most talked about, and these include dropping out of school, job loss, hospitalization, criminality, jail time and troubled relationships. Sometimes a person who is addicted does not seem to face these consequences of addiction but it is a progressive disease and eventually, even if someone is a functional addict, they will experience social problems if they don't get help for their addiction.

Spiritual Consequences

This type of consequences includes feeling hopeless, lonely, scared, guilty, ashamed, dishonest and perpetually unhappy, and restless for no apparent reason.

The impact of Addiction on Family life

The funny thing about addiction is that one person uses, but the whole family is affected. Addiction is a selfish habit as one is using drugs or taking alcohol to satisfy their fleshly desires of either been intoxicated or as a matter of running away from the reality of emotional discomfort. People have entertained addictions for a long time even when it has directly put them in bad space with families. Otherwise, no parent, sibling or wife wants to see their loved one struggle with the burden of addiction. Addiction has a characteristic of self-deception in that the user is blinded to the negative effects even when they are evident. Family is one key support system in every one's life because family has always been there for us. Since day one, they bought diapers and probably even buy the coffin after we die. Families go through a lot of pain seeing their loved ones struggle and wasting away at the hands of the silent devil.

I have personally lost a lot of family and friends to addiction, some of them bread winners and pillers of society, others wives, mothers, husbands, brothers and sisters, addiction does not discriminate whether race or gender, it does not choose ones financial status whether rich or poor or no-matter how learned or ignorant one may have been. It's the silent devil that is ever awake, never asleep and patiently waiting to pounce on any individual who opens to fall victim to its doors.

Addiction strains relationships nomatter which person in the family has the problem. So it doesn't matter if it's a parent, child, spouse or sibling. Every member of the family struggles in the home. Some years back it took away a close mate of mine who was a medical doctor, he had graduated the previous year from a university abroad and come back to start his medical journey. Being a learned and medical expert, he understood the chemistry of medicines formulated to give desired feeling, so he stumbled across katermin, a drug that is used in the theatre to administer pain, and ease any feelings of discomfort similar to the same effects of lucrative drugs. He went deep into the drug, at first he started as a social user, using for the fun of it. Then the reasons why he was using changed over time, it become a way of coping with stress and negative emotions. Being within the medical framework, he had easy access to the drug without anyone suspecting his use. He thought he had it under control but his consumption gradually increased.

 From being a regular user, he built up a tolerance which required him to increase the dosage. This time came when he had issues with his family about his choice of girlfriend, his family perceived their relationship as toxic and somehow rejected the love of his life while the feelings were also mutual from the girlfriend's family as they also perceived their relationship as toxic, hence rejected him. This rejection further threw him off into addiction as it widened the gap between him and family. He continued his usage and addiction started having a grip on his health as he lost weight dramatically because it took away his appetite and his continued usage again which landed him in a fatal accident, almost costing his life. He was recklessly driving at high speed under the influence of drugs and alcohol, he then blacked out on the wheel and the car ran into a drainage over-turning three times. He woke up on a hospital bed in the Intensive Care Unit. Some months later, he checked into rehab and we sat and talked about the challenges we anticipated, and on that day, I remember he said the easy access and availability of drugs is what I fear most because as much as I am a doctor, this thing is beyond my control. He wanted to do away with the drug but his work place was the major trigger because he had full access to the drugs, this was a major stumbling block to his recovery. After being out for a month, it was just within days and he was back on the drug.

Many people recovering from harder drugs like cocaine and heroin and even codeine have this belief that alcohol is more manageable than the former drug of their choice, so they opt to shift to alcohol forgetting that alcohol impairs judgment. Many people slip back into their former drugs because whenever one is intoxicated with alcohol, the same sockets that make people crave for drugs are turned on if the drug is available, and this goes beyond choice and it's a subconscious push beyond the conscious mind. So for a start, one will say it was just a slip and wouldn't happen again. Many people have ended up relapsing and going back to their active use.

Family members also respond in different ways, some step back from the family unit to avoid engaging with the addict. They don't want to involve themselves with the chaos that come with addiction, while some will take the opposite role to try to influence or control the addict into stopping or getting help. Others take advantage of the situation to manipulate the addict for financial gain. I was also a victim of being taken advantage of and manipulated for others' financial gain. A few years ago I was an active user of marijuana and this was a time when addiction had taken over me and the only company of friends I kept were addicts. I became very careless and from my appearance, presentation and behavior, it was easy to pick that this person is struggling with some sort of substance. I was under the care of a close relative who never at any point confronted me about my drug use.

I returned home that day from my weekly squash training only to be received with news that two officers from the Drug Enforcement Commission had passed by home asking for my where abouts, and when asked why, they said I was being suspected of running a syndicate that was cultivating hundreds of acres of cannabis and I was needed to be tested at the Commissioner's office. The trick behind the story was that if my test results came out positive, I was going to be convicted, so lawyers were needed who were more conversant with the law. Huge sums of money were sent to pay for the legal fees when in reality there wasn't even a case but it was just a scam to extort money from the family, because obviously no parent would love to see their child being sent to jail. I was made to go through fake traditional rituals for protection at the hands of fake witch doctors. The truth was, I was a very active user of marijuana and my team never ran out of supplies, but I had no capacity to cultivate even a garden of marijuana, so many people have been manipulated and taken advantage of.

Children living with a single parent who abuses drugs do not have anyone else to turn to. This is not the same for children living in a two-parent household with both parents struggling. When only one parent has the problem though, there is another parent to step in, they still feel the effects of addiction but still have some support.

Children who live with an addicted parent grow up in unpredictable environment, their home is often filled with secrecy and role reversal. They receive inconsistent emotional and physical support. There is a much higher possibility of abuse or violence against these children.

I have personally seen families crumble at the expense of alcohol and drug addiction, a few years ago, I lost a close friend of mine a.k.a Bashi Kabwe, who took his life by drinking a concoction of bols whiskey, a pesticide called doom, and chlorine after his wife, who was also alcoholic, publicly cheated on him and threatened to leave him for her new boyfriend taking with her their two beautiful kids who were six and four years of age. He thought his world was ending because he couldn't imagine a life without the woman he loved so dearly and just the vision of another man sleeping with his wife and taking care of his kids was bit painful. Little did we know that he had gone into depression and was already contemplating suicide. On this fateful day, I was awakened by his two kids while on my routine afternoon nap in preparation for my night shift job as a security guard.

The kids burst into my one roomed shack screaming uncle Bwalya, mummy is asking for you, come see what Daddy has done. I ignored the call as it was an everyday thing for them to fight, but within a few minutes later, I got disturbed by a noisy crowd. I immediately rushed to my neighbor's house only to find shi-Kabwe spread out on the floor struggling for his breath with a white discharge coming out of his mouth, we tried to resuscitate him by offering immediate first aid, we mixed charcoal and salt to try and neutralize the concoction of pesticide he had drunk in an attempt to kill himself. His condition worsened and it became another case of brought in dead as they reached the hospital. The decision he made to take his life was a selfish one because he never thought about his kids, but I would be right to say this decision was made under the influence of alcohol which has been known to impair one's judgment.

We have witnessed people being divorced even after being married for 20 years plus, but still move on. Even the lifestyle and the home environment was very toxic because their lifestyle was characterized by alcohol abuse. The dysfunction in the family was very evident in that their marriage was an abusive one.

2

Recovery And Sobriety

Recovery means healing. Sobriety just means being sober or abstaining from drugs or alcohol. Recovery is learning to love ourselves and others. Recovery is finding peace. Recovery is continually becoming a better person. Recovery is owning up to our actions right or wrong and giving up the victim role. Recovery is making amends, and not just saying we are sorry. Recovery is action. Recovery is daily. Recovery isn't a one- time thing, it is a lifelong journey.

Sober or clean – means just that. You are physically sober and clean.

Recovery is much more than just putting substances down. Anyone can put the drugs and drink away for a day and call themselves sober, but not everyone can say they are in recovery. Not everyone can say they have begun the journey to better themselves. Whatever it is you are doing to make yourself better each day, whatever you are doing to put the person you were while using, is in recovery. You are healing. You are getting better.

Recovery offers you a lifelong, wonderful experience of getting to give you your best shot every day. Life isn't just about not using on a daily basis, it is about having the human experience that is living as well. Of course, recovery wouldn't be possible if you were not sober first, so staying sober is one of the most important factors for recovery, but it isn't the only one. Recovery is an individual experience of getting better.

It is the restoration of a person to his normal functioning and reasoning without using drugs or substances.

Recovery may mean different things to different people, recovery also means self-discovery because it is a process by which one rediscovers themselves becoming aware of their thought patterns, emotional management, healthy stress coping skills and one also becomes more aware of their strengths as well as weaknesses.

Recovery begins when one acknowledging and accepting that they have a problem and it is beyond their control hence opening to learn about the root cause of one's problem and also learn how to create a life that is easy to live every day without resorting to substances use as a way of coping. I took time to dedicate and honestly explore more about my personality, what am capable of, and what areas I needed to focus on and many of us who had hit rock bottom took and embraced recovery as a second chance to make it right with life.

Understanding addiction can be complicated enough, but getting sober can seem like you are learning a new language entirely. You may hear some say they are sober while others say they are in recovery or recovered. But still others will refer to themselves as an alcoholic or an addict. But what does that mean? It depends on who you ask. How should you refer to yourself when you stop using drugs or alcohol? They are likely as many answers to that question as the people you ask, and in the end, it's a personal decision.

For those who started using drugs or alcohol early in life, recovery might be more of discovery of a state of health or mind without using substances.

One of the most interesting aspects of being in recovery is that there is no time requirement and no time limit. If you commit to stop using drugs today, you are in recovery, likewise, if you quit using drugs twenty years ago, you are still in recovery.

Recovery is an ongoing process and lasts as long as you are living, hence the phrase recovery suggests a lifelong process. No matter how long one abstains from substances, they never become immune to their triggers. These never change size or color. Triggers will always be triggers and the best and only response to one's triggers is to avoid them. Triggers may differ from individual to individual, because what might trigger me may not trigger the next person. Hence, my understanding that recovery from addiction is not like recovering from an illness like malaria where one is prescribed a course of medicine, but recovery is everything from introspection of one's lifestyle to continuously striving and improving your life. Another interesting part of being in recovery is that it can be called so many different things. There are so many ways to describe your recovery from drugs and alcohol. Here are just a few examples of how you might describe yourself.

> I 'm in recovery
> I 'm an addict in recovery
> I 'm clean and sober
> I 'm a recovered addict
> I 'm a recovering addict

The beauty is that all these statements add up to the same thing as long as you are not using and you get to choose. It is part of owning your recovery.

Recovery is a process of change through which people improve their health and wellness, live self-directed lives, and strive to reach their full potential. Even people with severe and chronic substance use disorders can, with help overcome their illness and regain health and social function. This is called remission. Being in recovery is when those positive changes and values become part of a voluntarily adopted lifestyle. While many people in recovery believe that abstinence from all substance use is a cardinal feature of a recovery lifestyle, others report that handling negative feelings without using substances and living a contributive life are more important parts of their recovery.

Addiction is considered a brain disorder because it involves functional changes to brain circuits involved in reward, stress, and self-control. These changes may last a long time after a person has stopped taking drugs.

Those functional changes to the brain and the long lasting nature of it, even after you've quit using, are what color the difference.

The state of sobriety is momentarily and passive in a way while recovery is the active process of staying sober. One that requires diligence, constant attention to your state of mind, situational awareness, and continuous work on addressing the underlying cause of your initial substance use disorder.

Recovery is the journey of staying sober and achieving long lasting sobriety.

From achieving sobriety to recovery

Achieving sobriety takes commitment and effort. The first thing is deciding you want to change your life and fix the addiction that controls you. You need to look back recognizing the need and want to live a life that you are in command of as a pivotal moment in your life. This is when the journey towards sobriety begins. To achieve it in a literal sense, you need to go through a detox which is your body's natural process of ridding itself of the chemicals you've been putting, be it alcohol or drugs.

It is recommended to do this at a treatment center as detoxification can lead to potentially severe withdrawal symptoms- your body and mind have grown accustomed to functioning with drugs or alcohol. As such, withdrawing throws your system out of work, so 24/7 care and attention ensures you get through them as comfortable as possible. At that point, by definition of the word, you are sober.

But because you haven't worked through the root issues that led you to take substances, your sobriety is extremely fragile and any inconvenience or problem that arises which you're not ready for, big or small, can trigger a relapse.

This is where the active work of recovery comes to support your newly won sobriety.

Depending on your addiction and how serious it was, it's highly advised that you attend some type of treatment, since detox isn't a solution by itself. For less severe substance use disorders, outpatient care is generally suitable, whereas, for heavier addictions, in-patient care is more effective.

Rest assured though, no matter which rehab center you choose, each person is assessed on an individual basis, and recommendations are made according to that.

With rehab, you truly dig into the causes of your addiction and develop a new, healthy coping mechanism to use in place of substances, with treatment centered on talk therapy in both individual and group settings that serve as a foundation for sobriety.

The difference between inpatient and outpatient care is that with inpatient care you live at the facility and thus it is more regimented and controlled, hence it is recommended for those with more severe addictions.

Once you finish rehab, participating in aftercare is how you maintain that sobriety you have worked so hard to achieve.

There are several myths and misconceptions that surround addiction and keep many people who suffer from telling others about what they are going through. One struggle includes the social stigma that often surrounds addiction. People often hesitate to tell their families and friends for fear of being criticized or abandoned. The best thing people can do for someone in recovery from an addiction is stand by their side during ongoing journey. Recovering from an addiction is difficult when done alone. Even after treatment, it is important for people to understand what one endures while being addicted. That way families, friends and spouses can band together to help the person in recovery stick to the sobriety plan.

Setbacks in recovery

When people start thinking about quitting drugs and alcohol, they often imagine that recovery is only about abstinence. They believe that they will be fine as long as they can resist drinking or using again.

However, they soon discover that there is a lot more to recovery. They encounter many unexpected challenges, and some of the biggest challenges are the tricks played by their own minds. The following are some of the most common challenges people encounter during their first year of recovery from addiction;

Difficult Emotions- for many people, staying sober isn't terribly difficult as long as life is going pretty smoothly and they are in a pretty good mood. Unfortunately, few of us get to abide in such a care free state for long. Problems arise, bad things happen, and sometimes we just feel bad for no apparent reasons. Dealing with difficult emotions is one of the biggest recovery challenges because drug and alcohol use often begin as a way of coping with these kinds of emotions. Stress is perhaps the biggest culprit but shame, anger, grief, sadness and anxiety are major challenges as well. One of the most important parts of addiction recovery is learning strategies to manage stress and cope with challenging emotions.

Cravings- you might predict that cravings would be a problem when recovering from addiction since you no doubt experienced plenty of cravings during active addiction. However, coping with cravings when you intend to never use drugs and alcohol again is a next level challenge because you often experience a craving as a sort of command that's very hard to refuse. Learning to deal with cravings takes a multi-faceted approach that includes identifying and avoiding triggers, behavioral strategies to keep from giving in to a craving, and emotional regulation strategies such as distraction, surfing the craving, and staying present.

Relationship Problems- your health and your career can survive addiction for a little while, but your relationships are usually the first to suffer. Substance use quickly leads to deceptive behavior, which undermines trust in a relationship. Your priorities become focused on drugs and alcohol and you neglect your responsibilities to your friends and family. You may even get to a point where you are lying to them or stealing from them to feed your addiction. Drugs and alcohol impair your judgment, leading to more fights and faster escalation, and the list goes on. On the other hand, social support is one of the most important things in recovery. A lot of sober people find themselves examining burnt bridges, wondering which ones can be repaired.

Money Problems- after relationships, addiction is almost always hard on your finances. Drugs and alcohol cost money, some drugs cost a lot of money. However, the really crippling expenses are secondary. They include high interest debts, legal and medical costs and lost income. It can be pretty demoralizing to come out of a treatment, feeling like you have made a pretty good start turning your life around, only to realize your finances are in total chaos. It can certainly adds to the stress discussed above. These problems can be overcome and they are certainly easier to overcome when you are sober, but it will take time.

Loneliness- people starting out in recovery often face a dilemma, they know that if they spend time with old friends who drink and use drugs, they will likely slide back into old habits, but they have not yet made new friends and so they often feel lonely. Loneliness itself is often a challenge because it can lead to boredom, depression, and anxiety, which are not helpful for recovery. As noted above, social connection is an especially important part of recovery. So loneliness is nothing to take lightly. Typically, the best way to deal with loneliness is to make friends within your recovery community. These can be people you went through treatment with, people from your 12 step group. These are people you see regularly, who understand what you have been through and share commitment to sobriety.

Boredom- people are often surprised how big of a challenge boredom is in recovery. There are two reasons boredom is so powerful. First, drugs and alcohol take up a lot of your time. You have to get them which sometimes takes some effort, and you have to carve out enough time to use them with the least amount of trouble. When people quit, they suddenly find they have loads of free time and they are not sure what to do with it.

The second reason is that addiction actually restructures your brain. Drugs and alcohol become the most interesting things in the world and everything else is a bit dull by comparison. Drugs and alcohol can also enhance your experiences, so even things you liked to do that were not substance related might suddenly seem flat. Again, coping with this is a matter of deploying smart behavioral strategies and to some extent just being patient while your brain adopts to sober life.

Mental Health Issues- the majority of people with substance use issues have concurring mental health issues. A quality treatment program will identify and begin treatment of any mental health issues, since managing them is essential to a long recovery. However, people who try to get sober on their own or by going to AA or NA meetings might find that getting sober throws their mental health issues into sharper relief. Often, some form of therapy is necessary if recovery is going to last.

Transitioning Home- transitioning from a treatment facility back to normal life is often more challenging than people realize. They go from a highly structured, sheltered, and supportive environment back to basically the same environment where their drinking and drug use was out of control. There is a big difference between coping with a problem in a controlled environment and coping in real life. For that reason, transitional care is very important. This might take the form of stepping down to a lower level of care such as an intensive outpatient program, a sober living environment, or transitional services.

Addiction recovery is a lengthy process that requires more than just mental toughness and plain old dedication. The journey to staying clean is full of setbacks and pitfalls which, if not overcome, often lead to a relapse. Staying clean is a lifelong commitment.

If you haven't experienced having a substance use disorder, recovering from one may seem like an easy task. Admit you have a problem, ask for help, receive professional treatment, get sober, and then stay sober. However, anyone that has an addiction or has witnessed a loved one go through treatment will tell you otherwise. Addiction recovery setbacks will happen, often recovery is not a linear journey.

People in recovery can falter after a period of sobriety. This is called a relapse or a recovery road block, and it can cause feelings of disappointment. While a setback like this can seem like failure, it is an extremely common part of recovery. Up to 60% of people recovering from substance use disorder will relapse within their first year of treatment. The chance of going through an addiction setback is something people in recovery live with daily.

As someone who is going through addiction treatment, you may be attracted to risky behavior patterns that are attached to having a substance use disorder. Long-term recovery is only possible only if you recognize these patterns and learn how to avoid them along with substances you are likely to abuse.

Along with getting professional help, you may also need to cleanse your life completely of anything that causes a recovery roadblock, such as certain friends. If your addiction was condoned by some people, being in their presence might not be safe for you. While these friends can be supportive of your recovery and happy that you are doing better, they might not help you recover.

If you have struggled with addiction for a long time, some family members may have developed some enabling behaviors. These can be harmful and conflict with what you have learned in addiction treatment programs. You may also need to clean your environment and remove anything that will remind you of your addiction. Make sure you are not hoarding alcohol or drugs anywhere.

For most addicts, the fear of a relapse is always present. Coping with the temptations of substance abuse, remaining sober and clean is a daily struggle. The recovering process involves a lot of aspects that starts with lifestyle changes. Lifestyle changes are a must do. Observing the same routines from your old lifestyle often leads to a relapse to the same habits.

A recovering opiate addict has to learn to build their new lifestyle around recovery. A holistic lifestyle change addresses the physical, mental, social, emotional and spiritual aspects of improving the odds of successful healing. No matter how daunting or hard it may get, it is of utmost importance to stick to the recovery process. A life of sobriety is a day to day living.

Some lifestyle changes include embracing honesty, addicts live in a lie that one is okay while they are not. Being honest with yourself and even to family and friends allows one to accept that all is not well and that you need help. If you find yourself lying to others, you are more likely to slip back into addiction and need to evaluate your standing. When it comes to your recovery struggles, do not lie about it and more importantly, never lie to your sponsor. Be accountable for your actions.

Our friends and hobbies can be our enablers. A recovering addict should not be around people who are still using. New hobbies take up time and money previously spent on substance abuse. New friends and hobbies help recovering addicts to reconnect with what they are missing because when one is in active addiction, it takes up all their time and even money because it is of main focus, so recovering addicts now tend to have a lot of free time and even money at their disposal because there is now this void left by the absence of addiction. Rekindling relationships and rebuilding trust with friends and family members who are supportive of your recovery can help a recovering addict live a new fulfilling life.

3
What Is A Relapse?

Our bodies and brains are wired to repeat activities that we find pleasurable. After years of repeating a behavior over and over again, a behavior that triggers the *feel good* hormone in the brain called dopamine, it is very likely to have us to fall back into the same old pattern, and at some point drugs and alcohol become the main source of this dopamine. This happens with drug or alcohol abuse. Repetitive substance use is something our body gets used to, becomes reliant on, and continues to crave even after the drugs have stopped. When someone gives in to these cravings after they have been sober or in rehab, it is considered a relapse. Relapse is one of the scariest words in recovery, but it is also a very normal part of recovery process especially for those in the early adjustment stages.

A relapse is a worsening of a clinical condition that had previously improved

In addiction treatment, relapse is the resumption of substance use after an attempt to stop, or a period of abstinence. For example someone who returns to active alcohol or drug use after months in rehab would be experiencing a relapse.

It is important to know that relapse is possible, and often a very normal part of the recovery process. While relapse is very common in recovery for some drugs, it can be very dangerous and lead to overdose.

A relapse happens when a person stops maintaining his or her goal of reducing or avoiding use of alcohol or other drugs and returns to previous levels of use.

Recovering from a dependence on alcohol or another drug is a process that can take time. A relapse happens when a person stops maintaining their goal of reducing or avoiding use of alcohol or other drugs and returns to their previous levels of use.

This is different from a lapse, which is a temporary departure from a person's alcohol and other drug goals followed by a return to their original goals. For example, a person who has set a goal of not drinking alcohol may end up having a glass of wine at a party, only to return to their alcohol goal the following day.

The degree of substance use can vary within a lapse, but what makes a lapse different from a relapse is that it is a brief period of substance use followed by a clear return to the person's recovery goals.

What causes a relapse to happen?

Many things can lead a person to relapse. There is a strong connection between dependent alcohol or other drug use and personal challenges. These can cause problems at work, on-going emotional psychological issues, and social or economic problems such as financial hardship, rejection by social support and challenges in personal relationships.

A relapse is not a sign that a person is weak or a failure, it's just a continuation of old coping patterns that need to be replaced with new ones.

Contrary to popular belief that a relapse is quick, almost situational occurrence, it is actually a slow process that occurs in three stages; emotional, mental and physical. Being aware of these three stages can help prevent relapse.

Relapse is a process rather than an event, it starts in subtle ways and increasingly gets worse. In order to understand prevention, one must understand the stages of relapse.

Stage 1- Emotional relapse: this is the first phase of the three phases of relapse. During this stage, the person is not actively thinking about using drugs or alcohol. However, their emotions and behaviors may be setting them up for a relapse down the road. Some of the signs of emotional relapse include:

Bottling up emotions, not going for recovery support meetings

Isolating yourself from peers and family

Going to meetings and not sharing

Focusing on other people and their problems to avoid your own

Not managing anxiety, anger, or other emotional problems in a healthy way

Intolerance

Defensive

Mood swings

Not asking for help

Poor self-care emotionally or physically

Not having sober fun or taking time for yourself

To prevent getting stuck in the first stage on the road to relapse, it is helpful to ask yourself some questions to gain awareness through self-reflection. Try asking yourself the following self-reflection questions:

Are you being good to yourself?

How are you having fun?

Are you putting time aside for yourself, or are you getting caught up in life or drama of others?

Which coping skills are you using?

What can you add to your recovery program to keep you in a safe place emotionally and physically?

Are you addressing your emotions, feelings and thoughts? If not, why not?

Have you been attending and participating in recovery support meetings?

How are you managing stressors?

Can you compare your self-care and behaviors now with the way they were when you were actively using? What is similar, and what has changed?

To prevent relapse, it is crucial to recognize that you are in emotional relapse and seeking to immediately change your behavior. If you are feeling anxious, begin implementing deep breathing techniques.

Denial is very common in the emotional relapse stage. When one has been in emotional relapse for a period of time, they begin to feel uncomfortable or not at ease in their own skin. This results in feeling discontent, restless and irritable. Unfortunately, due to fear of judgment or failure, many do not share how they are feeling when this occurs. However, sharing how you are feeling is crucial at this stage. If you don't begin practicing self-care, you become exhausted, when you are exhausted you want to escape. As tension builds, one becomes at greater risk of moving into stage 2-mental relapse.

Stage 2: Mental Relapse- When we choose to not work on any signs or symptoms of the emotional stage, there is increased risk of transitioning to the second stage of relapse, which is mental relapse. Once in mental relapse, which is best described as a war going on inside one's mind, the individual is at high risk of physical relapse. Part of them wants to use while the part doesn't. Fantasizing about using is not uncommon in this stage. As individuals go deeper into mental relapse stage, their cognitive resistance to relapse diminishes and their need of escape increases. It is important to remember that occasional thoughts of using are normal in early recovery.

The signs of mental relapse include:

Cravings or physical and psychological urges to use drugs or alcohol

Thinking about people, places, and things associated with past use

Hanging out with old friends who use alcohol or other drugs.

Minimizing consequences of past use or glamorizing past use

Bargaining

In bargaining, individuals start to think of scenarios in which it would be acceptable to use. A common example is when people give themselves permission to use on holidays or visiting family.

Another form of bargaining is when people start to think they can relapse periodically, perhaps in a controlled way, for example, once or twice a year.

Bargaining can also take the form of switching one addictive substance to another.

- Lying
- Thinking of schemes to better control using
- Looking for relapse opportunities (hanging out with old friends or missing meetings)
- Imagining using
- Fantasizing about using
- Planning your relapse
- It is important to remember that it gets harder to make the right choices as the pull of addiction gets stronger.

Techniques for dealing with mental relapse include:

Play the tape through

When you think about using, it is easy to believe that you are able to control your use this time. Imagine the consequences of what will happen, whether physical, psychological, or other, and decide if it is really worth it. You may not be able to stop the next day, and you will get caught in the same vicious cycle.

Talk to a trusted peer

A helpful tool is expressing your thoughts and feelings with a trusted friend, family member, or member of a support group. As you begin to share your thoughts and feelings, your urges begin to dissipate. They won't feel so overwhelming, and you will feel less alone.

Wait for 30 minutes

Most urges usually last approximately 15 to 30 minutes max. It may feel like an eternity, but if you keep yourself busy or distract yourself, it will quickly diminish. Taking a 30 minute walk is also very helpful.

Take it one day at a time

Try not to focus on whether you can stay abstinent forever. For now, take it one day at a time to become productive and take time to focus on yourself.

Use relaxation techniques

Relaxation is an important tool in relapse prevention. This is because when you are tense, relaxation techniques help reduce tension.

Stage 3- Physical Relapse

When a person doesn't take time to acknowledge and address the symptoms of emotional and mental relapse, it doesn't take long to lead down the path to physical relapse. This includes the act of drinking alcohol or using other drugs. The key is to reach out for help if you find yourself in physical relapse immediately in order to stop the vicious cycle of addiction before it is too late.

Causes of relapse

Recovery from alcohol or other drugs is a process of personal growth with developmental milestones. At any stage of recovery, there is a risk of relapsing, making relapse prevention skills highly important to know and understand. Some of the most common triggers of relapse include;

- Boredom
- Stress
- Money problems
- Relationship issues
- Certain sights and smells
- Certain people or places
- Falling into old habits
- Anger
- Insecure housing, professional or personal setbacks, social pressures or social stigma.
- Pre-existing mental health or emotional issues.
- Pre-existing physical health issues. Poor physical health can cause some people to use non-prescription pharmaceutical drugs, particularly when they have persistent pain.
- Guilt caused by lapsing. A person trying to abstain from substance use can experience internal conflict or guilt if they end up lapsing. If not managed properly, this situation can lead to self-blame and guilt that in turn mean the person is more likely to continue.

Long-term solutions for managing relapses are about preventing relapses as much as possible, same as long recovery is about creating a life that is easy not to use drugs or alcohol. This life can only be possible in the absence of your triggers.

Avoid certain people places and things

Steering clear of people, places and situations that used to lead the person to use alcohol or other drugs.

Self-care and a balanced lifestyle

Not taking care of yourself physically and mentally can be a trigger for substance use. One should be encouraged to adopt healthier lifestyle behaviors like getting enough sleep and time for recuperation, eating nourishing food and having a clean living environment.

Thinking differently

Along with the person's short term goals of reframing the way they see events, encourage them to try to learn from their mistakes, build a positive self-image and set future goals, including goals unrelated to their alcohol and other drug use.

Relapse Prevention

There are four main ideas in relapse prevention. First, relapse is a gradual process with distinct stages. The goal of treatment is to help individuals recognize the early stages, in which the chances of success are greatest. Second, recovery is a process of personal growth with developmental milestones. Each stage of recovery has its own risk of relapse. Third, the main tools of relapse prevention are cognitive therapy, mind-body relaxation, which are used to develop healthy coping skills.

Most people who struggle with addictions are blind to its negative effects. Deception is a characteristic of addiction where the one using is overlooking the negative impact even when the negative effects of health may be life threatening. I personally had a rough ride full of heart breaking experiences where my life was very stagnant in terms of making decisions, life progressive decisions! I chose a path of self-destruction characterized by excessive alcohol use disorder which landed me in problems. In one incident, I started work as a security guard under Group 4 Security Company at Kansanshi Copper and Gold Mine, this was a time I was struggling with unemployment and the order of the day was just waking up and planning on how we would find alcohol to get us through the day.

My friend Antony who had travelled to Solwezi earlier that year informed me that there was an opportunity in Solwezi where a local contractor was employing over 500 electricians. I immediately organized transport and packed my bags and left for Solwezi. I arrived in solwezi and was received by my friend who had offered to accommodate me at his cousin's place. I was taken to Freca's office, the contractor who was said to be hiring. I found thousands of people from all walks of life hoping to get a job. I waited with the crowed for a while then picked up the courage to approach the humans resource only to be told that they had recruited the last batch of electricians the previous day. My friend advised me to stay for a while and look out to other opportunities. A few days later, I was rejected, my friend's cousin told to me find an alternative place to stay because he complained that he couldn't keep two grown unemployed adults. I approached a friend of ours who was running a business of assembling pool tables on behalf of his nephew who was on the Copperbelt. This friend by the name of Brain used to sleep right there in the shop.

I explained to him what had transpired concerning the place where I was being accommodated. He agreed to stay with me in the shop as until I found a job and could rent a place of my own. I started helping him out at the shop assembling pool tables and servicing juke boxes. My friend stumbled across an advert in which Group 4 Security Company was recruiting guards to work at the mines with minimum qualification being a grade nine school certificate. I got engaged into this job as a security guard at the mines. I started working night shifts at an isolated crasher, where it was very rocky, dusty and my job was to control who had access to this location and make sure they were abiding by the safety regulations. Because the place was very cold and usually with minimum activity at night, I started carrying some marijuana and whiskey to help me get through the night.

This become a daily habit as I would team up with other guards from different sights and share weed and alcohol then go back to our locations. As time went by, I become so comfortable with this habit of smuggling weed and alcohol at work and getting intoxicated on duty. Some of my other colleagues noticed on this one occasion when I got so drunk and I carelessly flashed the alcohol bottles. Part of my frustrations which pushed me into this behavior was failure to come to terms with how a graduate from a university qualified in electrical engineering was doing this odd job as a security guard. In reality, I was experiencing some dissonance which me pushed into the drinking. The money aspect was an another point of frustration as it was barely hand to mouth and working to pay the money lenders called shylocks. The salary couldn't get me through the month, so in a quest of trying to compensate for this, I got introduced to stealing and concealing copper cables from a nearby dump sight.

We eluded our fellow security guards who manned the entry boom gates by carefully stacking the compressed copper wires in helmets and in our small bags. In that moment, I thought it was all fun and adventurous, never being aware that I was engaging in these criminal acts not to put food on the table but to fund my addiction. On this fateful day, I was knocking off from the night shift intoxicated as usual from the smuggled alcohol. I was called into our superior office to collect a bus pass. As I passed by the seniors sat in that office, one of them detected a strong smell of alcohol and immediately I was subjected to the alcohol detector which tested positive for alcohol. I was put on forced leave for two weeks after which I went for a disciplinary hearing which was just for formality, the decision had already been passed that I was being discharged of my duties because this wasn't my first offence. There was also an incident where I was caught trying to smuggle out boots and uniforms with intentions of trading them for cash.

The process of helping out someone with an addiction starts with making the person first point out how negatively it has affected them or help them reflect on the worst circumstances addiction put them through. This leads to one coming to a realization that the addiction is beyond their control and will also give a person reasons to want to do away with their addiction. Many people would be in denial and tend to reduce the impact of addictions hence finding every reason to justify their use. It's a process of trying to help out one reflect on their life and see if their substance use has played a negative influence on their progress in general. When one moves past the stage of denial and accepts that they have a problem, it becomes easier to look at what areas of their life has been hit badly and also can now formulate a treatment plan based on the complaints and specific areas of concern, but generally, recovery from addiction covers a number of areas.

Among the areas one needs to tackle are substance use triggers. A substance use trigger is something that makes you want to use drugs or alcohol again. A trigger can be anything that reminds you or causes you to engage in unwanted behavior like substance use, it can be a person such as a friend, a spouse or even a relative and usually these people can be considered as toxic people. It can also be a place where you have easy access to alcohol or drugs like bars or night clubs, or places which hub suppliers, an emotional trigger may be anger, sadness, frustration, depression or even excitement. Other triggers may be things like money which grant you easy access to substances or things like music which reminds you of past drug use. Certain situations may also pose as triggers like events which in the past were celebrated by using substances for example holidays or family gatherings or even birthdays.

So as addiction is a chronic progressive illness, the reasons why one will start will differ from why they continue to use. I chose to first smoke marijuana because my friends where doing it and out of curiosity, I wanted to experiment and fit in with the group. It then became an activity that we enjoyed and looked forward to. Then in the long run, it became a way of coping in different circumstances like whenever I was stressed, I resorted to coping with substances. So the triggers will change according to what stage one may be on and they also differ from individual to individual. When one becomes aware of their triggers, they are better placed to create a plan on how to avoid those triggers and also create a plan on how to react to those triggers when they cannot be avoided. Recovery also requires one to do an introspection which is a process that involves looking inward to examine one's own thoughts and emotions. The first step in the process of introspection, or self-reflection, is accepting the past.

A person needs to acknowledge that the behaviors they participated in while abusing a substance were a direct result of that addiction, and more importantly, that addiction was a symptom of something deeper. Once a person looks beneath everything, the harmful

behaviors and actions, the addictions and everything else and finds
the root cause of their addictions and the resulting behaviors, they
begin to work on all of it and heal themselves. Without this hard
work, long term recovery is almost certainly not possible.

The question that has been frequently coming up from most
recovering addicts is how to manage to live among your triggers and
not get triggered to going into relapse. When one has been
consistently working on themselves and has a clearly defined purpose,
it makes the journey much easier because after understanding the
power that you command over your life, the power of your internal
locus of control, you begin to understand that you can rise above your
environment. Rising above your environment entails that you do not
let your environment limit your thinking or restrict your plans. Your
external environment should not detect how you should feel or what
you should think and what you should do. This comes to having a
clearly defined road map to dreams and aspirations. Rising above your
environment is being surrounded by negativity but choosing to stay
positive.

Active addicts are also frequently consumed with denial, since the
only way they can convince themselves is to keep using, denial makes
self-reflection difficult and keeps active addicts from understanding
their true selves. Once addicts enter recovery, they have the
opportunity to peek inside their minds and explore their inner
thoughts. With the ability to look inward, recovering addicts can spot
when their life is losing control. People who are in tune with their
innermost thoughts can often recognize when those thoughts
become dangerous

To be successful in recovery, the addict needs to want something
different. They need to be unhappy with their current situation and
have a strong desire to live differently. Reflecting deeply and honestly

on current relationships in one's life can bring about great awareness around how a person is feeling and why they are where they are. It is important to look at how you allow your relationships to affect you and how you participate in them. Are your relationships supportive of your goals or are they unhealthy?

Relationships are a direct reflection of a person's internal climate. A big step in recovery is letting go of unhealthy relationships. In order to really understand the relationships you have with others, you have to take an honest look inside.

Being addicted to drugs and alcohol is very difficult thing to overcome, but with a lot of hard work, honesty, determination to do the right thing for yourself, it is not impossible to overcome. Going through recovery you will learn tools that will help you deeper work, taking an honest look within and acknowledging the deepest truths will allow you to regain control of your life and begin to live with authenticity and joy In sobriety.

An addiction does not form spontaneously overnight. Instead, it is the result of a long process of repeated substance abuse that gradually changes how an individual sees a drug and how their body reacts to it. This process is linear and has the same progression for every person, although the duration of each step in that progression can differ greatly depending on the individual, dosage and type of drug being abused.

Since this process follows a pattern, it is possible to break it down into stages of an addiction, starting from a person's first use and leading all the way to addiction itself. There are seven stages of addiction and understanding each stage and the behaviors associated with each is a valuable way to identify when someone is at risk of an addiction or has already developed one. As each stage progresses so as the dangers associated with the drug's use, as the ability to quit using becomes much more difficult.

The first stage is called initiation, during which the individual tries a substance for the first time. This can happen almost at any time in a person's life. The reasons a teenager experiments with drugs can vary widely, but two common reasons are because of either curiosity or peer pressure. The latter choice is made with intent of trying fit in better with a particular group of peers. Another reason that teenagers are more likely to try a new drug than most age groups is due to how the prefrontal cortex in their brain is not yet completely developed. This affects their decision making process, and as a result many teenagers make their choice without effectively considering the long term consequences of their actions.

Just because someone has tried a drug does not mean they are certain to develop an addiction. In many cases, the individual takes a drug out of curiosity, and then once that curiosity has been satisfied, stops use. This decision can also be impacted by other factors related to the drug's role in the individual's life such as drug availability, peer usage, family environment and drug history, and mental health such as conditions of depression and anxiety often encourage use. If circumstances align and the individual continues to take the drug, they may soon find themselves in the second stage of addiction.

The second stage is experimentation, at this stage the user has moved passed simply trying the drug on his own and is now taking the drug into different contexts to see how it impacts their life. Generally, in this stage, the drug is connected to social actions, such as experiencing pleasure or relaxing after a long day. For teenagers, it is used to enhance party atmospheres or manage stress from schoolwork. Adults mainly enter experimentation either for pleasure or to combat stress.

During stage two, there are little to no cravings for the drug and the individual will be making a conscious choice of whether to use or not. They may use it compulsively in a controlled manner, and the frequency of both options mainly depends on a person's nature and reason for using the drug. There is no dependency at this point and the individual can still quit the drug easily if they decide to.

The third stage is regular use, as the person continues to experiment with a substance, its use becomes normalized and grows from periodic to regular use. This does not mean that they use it every day, rather that there is some sort of pattern associated with it. The pattern varies based on the person, but a few instances could be that they are taking it every weekend or during periods of emotional unrest like loneliness, boredom or stress. At this point, social users may begin taking their chosen drug alone, in turn taking the social element out of their decision.

The drug's use can also become problematic at this point and have a negative impact on a person's life. For example, the individual might begin showing up to work hung over or high after a night of drinking alcohol or smoking marijuana. There is still no addiction at this point, but the individual is likely to think of their chosen substance more often and may have begun developing a mental reliance on it. When this happens, quitting becomes harder but still a manageable goal without outside.

The fourth stage is risky use where the individual's regular use has continued to grow and is now frequently having a negative impact on their life. While a periodic hangover at work or an event is acceptable for stage 3, at stage 4, instances like that become a regular occurrence and its effects become noticeable. Although the user may not personally realize, people on the outside will almost certainly notice a shift in the behavior at this point. Some of the common changes to watch out for in a drug user include borrowing or stealing money, neglecting responsibilities such as work or family, attempting to hide their drug use, hiding drugs in easily accessible places, changing peer groups and losing interests in old habits.

The fifth stage of addiction is dependency, at this stage the person's drug use is no longer recreational or medical, but rather is due to becoming reliant on the substance of choice. This is sometimes viewed as a broad stage that includes forming a tolerance and dependence, but by now, the individual should have already developed a tolerance. As a result this stage should only be marked by dependence, which can be physical, psychological or both.

For a physical dependence, the individual has abused their chosen drug long enough that their body has adapted to its presence and learned to rely on it. If use abruptly stops, the body will react by entering withdrawal. This is characterized by a negative rebound filled with uncomfortable and sometimes dangerous symptoms,that should be managed by medical professionals. In most cases, individuals choose to continue their use, rather than seeking help, because it is the easiest and quickest way to escape withdrawal. With some drugs, especially prescription medications, the individual may enter this stage through psychological dependence before a physical one can form. When this happens, the individual believes that they need the drug to be able to function like a normal person. Here the drug becomes a coping mechanism for trying times, and then extends to instances where it should not actually be necessary. For example, a patient taking pain medication may begin to over-medicate, as they perceive moderate pain as severe pain.

In either case, the individual takes the drug because they have come to understanding that they need it in some way to continue through life. Once this mindset takes hold, addiction is nearly certain.

The sixth stage is addiction, dependency and addiction are words that are used interchangeably, and though the words are similar and frequently connected in drug use, they are different. One of the biggest difference is that when a person develops an addiction, their drug use is no longer a conscious choice. Up until that point, it remains at least a shadow of one. Individuals at this stage feel as though they can no longer deal with life without access to their chosen drug, and as a result, lose complete control of their choices and actions. The behavioral shift that began during stage four will grow to extremes, with the user likely giving up their old hobbies and actively avoiding friends and family. The may compulsively lie about their drug use when questioned and are quickly agitated if their lifestyle is threatened in any way. Users, at this point, can also be so out of touch with their old life that they do not recognize how their behaviors are detrimental and the effects that it has had on their relationships.

Another term for addiction is substance use disorder, which is an accurate description because it is a chronic disease that will present risks for a lifetime. Even after a person quits using drugs and has undergone treatment, there will always be a danger of a relapse. This means one must commit to an entire lifestyle change, in order to maintain their life of recovery.

The Crisis stage is the seventh and final stage which is the breaking point in a person's life. Once here, the individual's addiction has gone out of control and now presents a serious danger to their well-being. It is referred to as the crisis stage, because at this point the addiction is at the highest risk of suffering or another dramatic life event. Of course while crisis is the worst scenario for this stage, there is also a positive alternative that fits here instead. Either on their own or as a result of a crisis, this is when many individuals first find help from a rehab center to begin receiving treatment. As a result, this can mark the end of their addiction, as well as the start of a new life without drugs and alcohol, that is filled with hope for the future.

The Hard Truth About Recovering From Addiction

For many people, a substance addiction was an intruder that encroached into every aspect of their lives. Those who've successfully recovered from an addiction worked hard to understand what led them to substance abuse, and how they can keep the addiction from invading their lives again.

Sadly there are many myths and misconceptions that surround addiction and keep many who suffer from telling others about what they going through. One struggle includes the social stigma that often surrounds addiction. People often hesitate to tell their families and friends for fear of being criticized or abandoned. The best thing people can do for someone in recovery from an addiction is stand by their side during a long journey.

Recovering from an addiction is difficult when done alone, even well after treatment. Its important to understand what their loved ones endures while in addicted. That way, families, friends, and spouses can band together to help the person in recovery stick to their sobriety plan.

Here are things that people in recovery wish they could tell others about their struggles with addiction.

They Didn't Choose To Become Addicted

Addiction is never a person's choice. Plenty of people develop an addiction by taking drugs prescribed by a doctor to treat a medical condition. Over time, prescription drugs change the way a person's brain functions. They might continue taking pills to feel normal and be able to get through the day. Before they know it, an addiction has formed and the person may begin craving higher dosages of the prescribed substance.

10 lessons of Addiction Recovery That Are Rooted in Psychology

Recovery from an addiction is much more than mere abstinence from a substance or a behavior. Abstinence can be, and usually is, a fundamental component of the addiction recovery process, but abstinence does not necessarily equate to recovery .Recovery is a process of change through which people improve their health and wellness, live self-directed lives, and strive to reach their full potential.

Through the addiction recovery process, people can drastically change and improve their physical health, mental health, spiritual health, financial health, relationships, parenting skills, career capabilities, and the trajectory of their general life. The possibilities are endless. But in addition to drastic life changes in all areas of life, recovery from addiction also teaches valuable lessons. Below are just a handful of important lessons that can be learned through the addiction recovery process that have psychological undertones.

Life Has Meaning and Purpose- Every individual constructs their own sense of meaning and purpose in their life. The feeling that life and purpose can come from a variety of areas, such as career, family, nature, or spirituality and religiosity, among others. Sobriety can often be a catalyst of one's sense of meaning and purpose in the world In a variety of ways, Be it by being a better parent, a better colleague, a better friend, a better worker, a better member of the community, having a better experience on Earth, and so on.

Furthermore, many individuals in recovery from addiction have found that their suffering during active addiction has led them to personal transformation, and in some instances their experiences are used to help others with similar struggles. Giving back is very important to many in recovery from addiction, and in many instances is central to their sobriety.

Having a sense of meaning and purpose in life is extremely important to one's general wellbeing and quality of life, impacting us physically, mentally, spiritually, financially, relationally, and every which way in between. Recovery from any illness such as addiction can be a great catalyst for finding one's meaning and purpose in life and is a valuable lesson in addiction recovery.

Self-Esteem Comes From Within – Self-esteem can be defined as one's attitude towards themselves. More specially, do they have a positive or negative view of themselves. Self-esteem is an extremely important component of mental wellbeing. Oftentimes individuals who are addicted are plagued by immense feelings of shame and guilt due to the rippling impact of their addiction on themselves and on their loved ones, leading to a negative sense of self. Furthermore, being unable to reduce the frequency of their addiction or stop altogether implies weak will, due to a combination of such factors, addicted individuals often have low self-worth.

In turn low self-worth often exacerbates one's substance use or addictive behavior. The individual finds solace in their addiction, as it tends to either distract or numb them from their feelings of inferiority and insecurity, and also serves to give a false sense of confidence. While all substances can serve purposes, certain substances (depressants) such as opioids (heroin) , alcohol and benzodiazepines do a particular good job of numbing emotional pain while other substances such as cocaine and amphetamine do a particular good job of providing a false sense of confidence.

Addiction recovery often naturally results in an increased sense of worth and self-esteem merely by being able to stop engaging in an addictive behavior and putting aside the compromising behavior that often coincide with addiction. Furthermore, addiction recovery teaches individuals to build their sense of worth and esteem by doing the right thing. Additionally, individuals in recovery from addiction are often able to rebuild their relationships, their careers, their health and other such important life areas that improve their sense of self-respect, confidence, and dignity. Such issues are often worked on with addiction professionals during the addiction treatment process.

Gratitude Holds Great Power – "A grateful alcoholic (addict) does not use" is a common phrase tossed around the addiction recovery community. Gratitude is frequently a key component of the addiction recovery process. Addiction recovery teaches that even life does not appear to be going your way there is always something to be grateful for. This is important because gratitude plays a fundamental

Motivation is the driving force behind every action, it's also a primary component of the addiction recovery process. When embraced motivation can drive us away from the chaos and destruction of addiction, steering us into clean and sober lives.

The first step in recovery is admitting that you have a problem, the second step is having the willingness to accept or get help. For many people recognizing that they are engaging in bad habits is not difficult, but finding the motivation to address their addiction can be tough. This especially true for functioning addicts, who, even if they think they have a problem, don't find it serious enough to seek treatment. So what exactly motivates an addicted person to recover?

Addiction is a life-long illness, so in recovery, there are two parts to motivation one to enter recovery and one to remain in recovery.

Having the right motivation is a key aspect in overcoming addiction. In order for motivation to be real, you must find the benefits of recovery to outweigh the costs.

One of the most powerful vehicles for the road to recovery is intrinsic motivation. This means that you are motivated to do something for yourself and for yourself alone. For example, you want to quit alcohol because your liver is showing signs of damage from drinking, and you want to improve your health for your own sake.

Studies show that people with intrinsic motivation are most likely to overcome their addiction because it is stronger and more lasting. People who forced into treatment are probably destined to a less successful recovery.

Personal values – for some people, having an external factor is necessary for motivation. This can be anything that matters to you, such as a significant other, career, or even a self-image.

If you find a role model, or someone you don't want to disappoint, this can be a great motivational factor. For example, if you are a dad, you may want to be a better person for your kids.

Losing things that matter – Some people don't take their addiction seriously until they are confronted. A boss may hint at being fired. While threats and ultimatums can lead to a successful recovery, for some people it is a wakeup call.

If you are a family or a friend of an addict and considering issuing an ultimatum, try to avoid threats, especially as they may backfire. Feelings of shame and blame rarely motivate an addicted person to recover. Instead, try to convince them that they should seek treatment on their own terms. Instead of "I 'm filing for divorce unless you stop drinking", "Your drinking is impacting my wellbeing and our children's development or will you consider getting help?"

Support – Many people with addiction have low self-esteem or are not happy with some aspects of their lives.

If you are dissatisfied with your life, an unexpected show of support may be just what you need to seek treatment. You may be surprised that your family wants you to get better for your own sake, but you should be open to accepting change when it is offered. A supportive environment may be one of the strongest foundations for lasting recovery.

The promise for the future – In certain situations, you may be motivated to get clean by an unexpected life event. A sudden change that can potentially transform your life for the better can be inspiring. For example, you may have a child on the way or you may have been accepted into your dream university.

Scary situations – the opposite is true as well. You may be confronted with a wakeup call due to your addiction. For example, you may have suffered an overdose, had a run-in with the law, or lost a lot of money at the casino.

Tragic event – wake up calls can also happen on a larger scale. Perhaps one of your parents just passed away, which makes you rethink your life. Or you were diagnosed with lung cancer after smoking for decades. Maybe your actions impacted on someone around you. You may decide to change after one event that brings you clarity on your addiction.

Rock bottom – Small or medium scale tragedies can help people realize that they are in trouble, or the guilt from which it can motivate them to change. However, this is not always the case. In some situations, the stress or guilt is only temporary, and before they it, are back to their old habits.

Rock bottom refers to a situation where you realize you cannot go any lower, and there is no doubt that something needs to change. The definition of rock bottom is different for each person, for example, you may overdose once and want to change. For others, even if they overdose, after a few days to recover, they can just using again. Ultimately, rock bottom is when you realize that you are at a dead end and have no choice but to get clean.

Why do people get demotivated?

Just as there are many reasons that motivate an addicted person to recover, you must also consider the other side. In order to maintain recovery, it is important to be aware of the pitfalls that await you.

High expectations – having unrealistically high expectations about treatment can lead to a near immediate loss of motivation in recovery. You may think that you may just need to detox and then you are done, but it is just the first step. Or you might find that treatment is more challenging than you thought, and taking longer than expected. If this is the case, you may be tempted to give up.

Anger and Emotions – Going through therapy can cause past problems to resurface and force you to deal with your underlying issues, which isn't easy for anyone. This may cause you to get angry with yourself and other people around you. Powerful emotions can trigger you to give up and return to your addiction.

Poor preparation- If you are not adequately prepared for living a sober life after treatment, you can easily fall back into bad habits. For example, what if you go to party where everyone is drinking? What if you get into a confrontation with your family? You must have adequate coping skills before you leave a treatment program.

Relapse – many people associate relapse with failure: this is not true. Emotional or mental relapse is quite common, and commonly happens when you romanticize your past use, and forget all the negatives that come with it. A physical slip can happen as well, making you question why you ever tried to get better in the first place.

Relapse is a fact of addiction – all the good reasons that motivate an addicted person to recover may not be enough. But don't fear – relapse is part of getting better, and can actually strengthen your long term recovery. It can even be motivating for some, inspiring them to try harder next time.

Tips to motivate an addicted person to recover – It can be challenging to find and keep motivation during recovery, but it is crucial in the long run. Here are some tips to helping yourself or someone you love find motivation to seek treatment.

1. List the Pros and Cons

Remember, a key motivating factor is that the cost must outweigh the benefits. Therefore, take time to make a list of all the pros and cons of maintaining the addiction.

2. Meet Other People

Go to a meeting, read stories about addiction and recovery, or look up inspiring quotes. This can serve as a warning for those who have not hit rock bottom, and as a reminder to never go back

3. Ask for Support

Support can be a major motivating factor for people. If you need help, your friends and family will likely help you find the strength you need to get better. Having the right support will also help you believe in yourself.

4. Imagine a Better Future

Create goals, and think of what your life will be like once you quit. Create both long term and short term goals so that you don't get overwhelmed.

Finding motivation after treatment

Motivation is just as important for those who have completed treatment and are currently in recovery. To maintain a positive outlook, remember to celebrate the small achievements and don't forget why you are here in the first place.

Recovery is a long term journey and will take time and effort. That is why little success must be celebrated. Acknowledge each day you have been sober, and make sure you are reminded of it every day. Over time, you will see how far you have come and that will motivate you to keep going.

Always remind yourself what motivated you to get into treatment in the first place. Remember your dreams, your failures, and keep inspiring items out as a reminder. If you have a role model or a person you don't want to disappoint, keep a photo of them close by.

Most importantly, no matter what got you into the treatment in the first place, find a reason to do it for your own wellbeing. At the end of the day, no one impacts your life more than yourself.

How Do You Stay Motivated in Addiction Recovery?

It is often said that recovery from an addiction is a marathon not a sprint. As in a marathon, there are plenty of opportunities to give up in recovery and the people who do well aren't necessarily the ones who come blasting off the start line, but the ones who can keep themselves going when they feel totally exhausted. There is no easy trick to staying motivated, but some of the following strategies might help.

Understand that Motivation Is Variable – you need to understand first that motivation is not some intrinsic quality and it is not something you can do equally well every day. Motivation is a skill and sometimes you can do it well and other times you just have to be content to make it through the day. The good news is that like any skill, the more you practice motivating yourself and creating the right conditions for motivation, the easier it gets.

Identify your core values – when you are trying to keep yourself motivated, it helps to have a clear vision of why you are doing what you are doing. Otherwise, you don't have much incentive to persist through tough times. While it may be hard to picture your perfect sober life, you can certainly identify some of your core values and how staying sober relates to those values.

For example, many people decide to get sober when they realize what their drinking and drug use is doing to their family. For those people, it's important to keep the value of the family clearly in front of them. You can do this in various ways, you might keep pictures of your family around you, where you can see them easily. You might periodically write about why family is important to you. Studies have found that this exercise called self-affirmation can help you make healthier decisions and improve your relationships.

Create Good Habits — Motivation goes up and down, therefore it is important to create structures in your life to hedge against the risk of relapse on low motivation days. Part of that structure is made up of healthy habits and routines. It typically takes about two months for a new behavior to become automatic, but after that the new behavior is on auto-pilot. The more healthier habits you create, the more odds are stacked in your favor.

Build a Great Sober Network — another big part of creating a structure that will keep you on track is creating a great sober network. This includes sober friends, supportive family members and friends as well as your therapist in your recovery. A sober network helps you in many ways, it helps reduce stress because they are people who will listen without judgment and who can offer advice and support. You have more resources to deal with any problems that arise and you feel a greater sense of accountability.

Find Ways to Cope with Doubt- Learning to deal with doubt is crucial for staying motivated because nothing will kill your motivation faster than listening to that little voice that ask , " why are you putting yourself through this? You are just going to fail anyway." In order to stay motivated you have to have a reasonable expectation of success. The problem is that it is hard to judge what is reasonable, especially when you are just starting out.

Take One Day at a Time — This may sound cliché, but it is a cliché because it works. If you think that you have to motivate yourself to keep going forever, it will feel exhausting. However, if you only think that you have to make it through the day or even through the hour,that typically feels more manageable. You can only act in the present moment, so if you can motivate yourself to not drink, to call your therapist, or whatever you need to do right now, that's really all you have to worry about, if you can do it today, you can do it tomorrow too.

Play the Tape – Finally in an emergency, you can always play the tape. This is where you think of the consequences of drinking or using again. Typically, when you have a craving, you are only imagining the immediate gratification of drinking or using again. Unfortunately, that gratification only lasts a short time and then you have to deal with the consequences of relapse.

Getting And Staying Clean – We tend to get serious about overcoming an addiction when we realize it is in our best interest to do so. Naturally, a variety of factors prompt the desire for change – personal well-being, awareness of long term negative consequences, employment status or family issues to name just a few.

Regardless of the reason, it takes a high level of internal motivation to stay clean in the long run, without that firm commitment, we are virtually destined to fall short

Seated at a shabbin , one Monday morning with the neighborhood seniors, we chatted and argued about the countries political senieral in the countdown to the elections that year. Some stoned MMD barley who also happened to be my landlord by the name of Mr Sibale was always for the Bwezani admin after been put in charge of the ward treasurery. He always took matters of politics personal and at one point threatened to divorce his wife whom he had been married to for 30 years over a comment she passed over the escalating school fees. His best friend the owner of the shabbin was a die-hard supporter of the PF then in opposition . As we sat that Monday morning drinking a carton of the local shake beer for breakfast I the youngest was being counseled on the choice of marrying the neighborhood females who were always first customers at the local alcohol joint which kept people wondering what time they swept their homes.

This behavior was very prevalent and common among Zambian women who spent 3 quarters of the day drinking either in shabbins or local tarvens with little children in their backs. Just a few years back in Solwezi, this local I had a stint with got jailed for manslaughter of a her friends baby who she had wrapped in a chitenge on her back but as she got drank forgot and squeezed the baby against the wall. We argued about the countries voting patterns which were tribally marginalized, the southern province being the opposition and northern the rulling while the their was always a tag of war in the other provinces. As always, this shake beer breakfast meeting was my normal everyday schedule since dropping out of copperstone university were I went on a drinking spree with my school fees and exam fees ending me back on the streets taking my frustrations on alcohol and always blaming the govt for not providing employment to the youths.

My survival was based on handouts from family abroad otherwise fending off piece works for my dially drinking habits as years went by living without meaningful cause. My life style was the wrong role model type got hooked into smoking marijuana at the age of sixteen. I later graduated to diazepam sleeping pills or a.k.a blue mash and eventually alcohol was now the order of every day. A friend of mine by the name of Antony appeared at scene with with a worksuit engulfed in bana kasokopio, a vanacular name for black jack which sticks to ones cloths whenever you make physical contact. This plant is more of a weed as it grows wildly in bushes in very common in this part of the world, in recent times its also been adopted as a vegetable prepared as ifisashi given a nickname of kanunka which is bemba phrase for smelling. Before he was asked why he was engulfed in banakasopio as if he had been chasing a snake in the grass, he narrated that in the morning while he was watering the crops at a small co-operative block they were running as a family, he came across a Mbelele, vanacular name for a Sheep feasting on their cabbages and tomatoes which they subsistently cultivated.

He quickly mobilized the farm assistant and they chased the sheep until they captured it and locked it in one of the chicken runs. He then came back home to seek guidance from the elders on what he could do about this sheep that had been savaging their crops. One of the seniors Mr. Sinkonde advised that there were only two options, one was to take the sheep to the nearest police and the other was to look for the owner so he would pay for the damage done to the crops. He went on to explain the situation to his father who was the overall overseer at the co-operative block and was advised similarly to hand over the sheep to the owner or the police. He then asked me to accompany him as I was idly sitting without a plan and for me it looked like an opportunity to maybe make some money for alcohol.

We then engaged into a door to door campaign in search of the owner who was to pay for the sins committed by the sheep in the garden, we covered a big perimeter to no success only at one time were we directed to this guy of Nigerian origin by the name Juma who was the only person known to have been rearing sheep. We went to his house and found him just as he was entering his yard, then asked him if there was any sheep missing from his flock which he went and counted and found all of them were in tacked. We then wonder what we could next as we had gone around the neighborhood without any one claiming ownership. We thought of the other option of reporting to the police but we ruled it out and considered the option as non-starter because this seemed like it would be a loss on our part as police have always been known to be good at capitalizing on evidence and converting it for personal use. We then analyzed our situation as we both had no money, driven by our ambitions of alcoholic cravings we started brainstorming about who would be the possible buyers of the sheep.

I then thought the only place we could find a large number of people of West African origin was the mosque. The closest mosque was at lubambe centre in parklands which was about an hours drive from nkana east. Having no transport we decided to risk the crime of killing ants by taking a long walk to our alcoholic freedom in search of a buyer. We arrived at mosque to a quick welcome from a charcoal black man casually dressed man clad in black glasses who enquired if he could be any help on whatever business we had. We explained to him that we were selling a sheep. He asked our source and where it was, we then explained that it was the last among the many we were rearing but most of them had been sold out. He got our numbers and requested we come with it then we could consider doing business. We went by the nearest super market close to the mosque and negotiated with the shop keeper to leave one of our phones as surerity in exchange for some money to use as transport.

We in turn bought some Junta whiskey and ciggarates then harried back to the farm yard to collect the sheep. We tied the sheep In between a log and carried it with the farm assistant. The phones kept ringing from the papa as to find out how we were. We finally got to the mosque and traded the sheep for half the money we had initially intended to sail. We left to get the phone we had left by the super market and equally split the money 3 ways between us. Just after splitting we bought some disposable castle beer and celebrated a successful business deal with each one going his separate way. I boarded a bus through town to buy some cheap liquor called Tujilijili which were packed in small sachets. I drank the night away as was always the trend whenever I had money not caring what I would eat at night. My friend had proceeded to go for work in the evening as a security officer where he worked for Group 4 security company. I woke up around 09:00 hours the following day with a terrible hangover courtesy of the cheap Tujilijili which I had in the night. I went to the nieghbourhood shabeen as was always the culture and routine to scavenge for people nursing hangovers, I found the usual pair of elders having a treat of the local shake beer for breakfast who enquired on how we had moved with the sheep the previous day. Just as I was about to start explaining, Tony popped up from the other side of the fence holding a broom of which I immediately assumed he had he was sweeping the yard.

He excitedly greeted me in the usual mafia salute and enquired if I had any change from the deal from yesterday to jump start the drinking, he then engaged me on the latest which had just happened a while ago when the papa we sold the Mbelele from the mosque called requesting us to go and help him slaughter sheep for some extra cash and the offals meaning the intestines and inside wastes. I for one considered the deal a non-starter as we had already harvested from the fruits we did not sow, Tony insisted we take advantage of the situation and get more as our harvest from yesterdays deal was almost depleting. I eventually submitted to going with the idea and went back home to gear myself for the bonus deal anticipating how we would grab the sheep by its hornes and slit its throat and get more money from the papa.

I got some knives from the kitchen rack and packed them into the back pack went got to Tony's place I found him with Noah, a friend of ours and a son of the local shabeen's owner who was born among the other boys we had nicknamed the Milon brothers because of they were five boys all troublesome and strong who would sometimes fight amongst themselves until the police would be called to break up the confusion, gossip had it that this behavior was genetically inherited from their father who potraid traits of once a frustrated youth . As he saw us prepare he inquired about our plan of which he got interested and accompanied us to the mosque. We arrived at the mosque and Tony phoned the papa who requested us to present ourselves just by the main entrance where we could easily spotted. As we stood there trying to figure out where papa could be coming from, then come a rude shock as Tony was grabbed by his belt and trouser's by the papa ordering the closest taxi to stop while identifying us as thieves, I then realized it was serious and for a second thought of running but the place was crowded and my instincts kept me under control knowing that we had not stolen so we would just tell the truth and be set free.

We all got into the taxi and as it sped off, the papa furiously stressed that we had crooked him but we insisted that we were not criminals and we only managed to convince him to take us to the people who had consificated the mbelele. To our surprise we approached a big mansion in the residential area of river side were we found the yard was a filled with suvs, mercidis, range rovers and the most happening cars during that moment. We were ushered into the yard only to be received by a group of wealthy looking papa's dressed in boubus with wine glasses who looked like they were having a feast. At the first instant of seeing us, they one who looked more of the general dramatically assumed we were the thieves and ordered the papa to search us if we had any valuable gadgets on us so that he could consificate them and trade them in order to recover his money, unfortunately the only phones we had were brick phones nicknamed Tujilijii because of they were the cheapest on the market. They then started speaking in Arabic of which we could not understand anything, my friend Tony tried to bargain for them to speak English which we could understand but the only word we could hear was police.

We then got into the car and within the five minutes we were trying to negotiate our freedom we arrived at riverside police station. We all got out the car and entered the police station, the Papa was the first one to speak complaining to the male and female constable at the reception that we had deceived him into buying stolen Mbelele, immediately we were ordered to pass behind the desk and remove our shoes and surrender any valuables we had on us whilest been promised to be clobbered if found with any illegal substances. We then routinely searched and a small pocket knife was discovered on me which arose suspicion almost got me into more trouble until I explained that it was used for cable stripping for my electrician job.

We were then charged with stock theft and thrown into the cells while our phones were consificated. We found about eight people in the cells one girl who was under witness protection for witnessing a murder of her boyfriend who was brutally beaten to death by an identified stalker who burst into the girls house accusing the boyfriend of making advances against his girl when there was no relationship between them, rumor was that the local thugs had been tipped of the boyfriend to this girl having collected money from the family house they had just sold and hence this plan was merely an act of aggrevated robbery. The girl narrated that on that evening of the murder, the girl was with the boyfriend who was now deceased in the house preparing supper when they heard a knock on the door.

As the girl went to attend to the knock, the identified stalker burst into the house and accused the boyfriend of having an affair with his girl and thus the confrontation broke into a fight with the stalker dominating the weaker boyfriend, the girl was powerless as she witnessed her boyfriend been treated to a good beating then was later pulled outside the house into the street where a gang was patiently waiting to pounce on the powerless individual. They brutally beat him up and took everything he had on him, and left him to die by the street corner. The girl had remained at her house as this was happening, only to be woken up by an angry mob in the morning who come with stones and tires threatening to burn down her house after her boyfriend's body was discovered by just near her house and people had seen them together at the market place of which people jumped to the conclusion that she might have had a hand into her boyfriend's murder. She was only rescued by the police from the angry mob who threw stones at the police land cruiser as it sped off, hence putting the witness in the police cells for her own safety and also as a state witness.

The other guy was a care taker for a house under construction who stole 2 pockets of cement and sold it together with the wheel burrow on which he carried them on. He was later apprehended at a bar after it was discovered that cement had gone missing hence launching a manhunt for him and another guy was there for assaulting his friend who he suspected of having an affair with his girlfriend. The following morning at about 07;00 hours an old lady, a middle aged woman, a young girl about 12 years of age and a man in his late thirties come to the reception. The old lady explained that they had bought the man for discipline, it was reported by the neighbors that they heard the girl scream throughout and suspected she was being raped. The old lady who was the grandmother to the girl explained that the girl did not go home the previous night and they were also skeptical about her were abouts and got worried only to see her return in the morning with bruises on her neck.

The police officer on duty asked the girl what had happened and she in turn explained that she had been locked up at the guy's house and he forced himself on her as he repeatedly raped her, it was at this point that he was thrown into the cells and joined us behind bars. The police officer then requested the family to immediately take the girl to the hospital for a urine and blood test in order for the doctor to give a proper report on the condition and extent of the damage done to the girl. The gentle man was charged with rape and defilement of a minor. Inside the police cells, the guy disclosed that under the influence of alcohol he had forced himself on the minor. It never clicked in his mind that the girl was under age as he blamed this behavior on the alcohol.

The guy emotionally broke down as he now come to terms with reality. He disclosed his real age as 35 years of age not as he had cheated to be 19 years of age upon being thrown into the cells. He also explained that he was also married with his wife been 8 months pregnant as he kept wondering what had come into him while he constantly blamed his behavior on the alcohol. It was a long night for me in the cells as I failed to sleep with my thoughts racing and smelling jail around the corner. I was allowed to make a phone call as I tried to lobby for financial help from family who also shunned this move for fear of it being a scam as I previously played up such a similar scam just to get some money to fund my addiction this time around just like the boy who cried lion no one would come out. We spent the night in cells with a police man at the reception who was sneaking out on intervals to drink the Tujili jili common alcohol brand.

My victories against addiction has been mainly due to the deliberate steps I have taken to re- invent myself on an individual capacity. I must admit I face the same challenges as any other addict or any person who has struggled with addiction, am neither immune nor much less protected. The first part of my journey that has made it easy for me is taking responsibility for my actions rather than playing the blame game. The second is accepting the fact that I attract whatever surrounds me by the person I have become. A few years ago I was surrounded by drug dealers, thieves, criminals, prostitutes and junkies not because of the environment but I attracted everything around me at that time because of the person I became. Today it is a different story because i am surrounded by very productive and future focused individuals not because of luck but by deliberately spending hours to bring out my best possible version and not running away from challenges but embracing them as I continue to make them part of my story in my reinvention into a brand.

Reinventing yourself means identifying patterns, values, or activities that no longer serve you and changing them for better options. It can involve external characteristics, like job I am also an electrician worked as a security guard, a spanner boy,a ndunker boy, a garderner, a call boy, a vendor and a land scaper, hobbies, appearance, relationships, and location. True reinvention also happens inside, in how you think and behave

Reinventing yourself is not a standard process with a specific textbook or map. It's important to view your own reinvention as a journey of self-discovery. Reinventing yourself is related to finding your ikigai, or your reason for being. One of the steps towards reinventing yourself is self-awareness. This means carefully assessing your situation and what you want to achieve, then deliberately laying the steps and towards achieving your long term and short term goals. The secret to turning your dreams into reality is called action, commitment and recommitment. I believe we all have our ideal version within us, we just need to clear out the cobwebs in our thinking or simply distinguish between reality and fiction within our own thoughts, i call it taking a step back from yourself and challenging the thinking patterns we have adopted over time which have not been helpful.

ABOUT THE BOOK

The Invisible Observer talks about my personal experiences as an addict and real life circumstances that I went through and many people can relate to as I struggled with addictions and I have also shared some dramatic experiences some of them negative and I now consider as necessary. I have also shared some experiences from my friends and family members with a hope that someone can pick a lesson or two.

This book as also guild to anyone who would like to know more about addiction as I have deliberately gone in depth to explain the different components involved in addiction as well as recovery.

Roosevelt bwalya kasonso is a qualified electrical engineer from Copperstone University, He is a Certified counselor from the University of Zambia in Psychosocial counselling and HIV management, Child counselling, Couple's counselling and Addiction counselling. He is currently practicing as a therapist and also training to be a life coach. He is also a trainer in life skills on a group and individual capacity.